Clinician's Guide to ADHD Comorbidities in Children and Adolescents

Joseph Sadek

Clinician's Guide to ADHD Comorbidities in Children and Adolescents

Case Studies

Springer

Joseph Sadek
Department of Psychiatry
Dalhousie University
Halifax
Nova Scotia
Canada

ISBN 978-3-319-45634-8 ISBN 978-3-319-45635-5 (eBook)
https://doi.org/10.1007/978-3-319-45635-5

Library of Congress Control Number: 2018951434

This Springer imprint is published by the registered company Springer Nature Switzerland AG
The registered company address is: Gewerbestrasse 11, 6330 Cham, Switzerland

I want to give my sincere thanks to my wife Dr. Irene Sadek and my children.

Dr. Joseph Sadek and Ms. Maryanne Sadek who were extremely supportive during the journey of producing this book.

I would like to take this opportunity to thank Professor Dr. Lily Hechtman

For her effort and expertise that she contributed in reviewing the entire book and for writing the foreword.

I also would like to sincerely thank the following reviewers who are child and adolescent psychiatrists who reviewed and edited the individual chapters:

Dr. Alexa Bagnell, MD, FRCPC. Head of the IWK Child and Adolescent Psychiatry division

Dr. Normand Carrey, MD, FRCPC

Dr. Gerald Gray, MD, FRCPC

Dr. Anita Hickey, MD, FRCPC

Dr. Suzanne Zinck, MD, FRCPC

It would be impossible to produce this work and maintain the high standards of publishing without their thoughtful, insightful, and scholarly evaluation and expertise.

Finally, special thanks to Ms. Maryanne Michelle Sadek, University of Ottawa, for her efforts in compiling the appendices and conducting numerous literature reviews.

Foreword

Dr. Sadek, who is a psychiatrist and associate professor in the Department of Psychiatry at Dalhousie University in Halifax, Nova Scotia, has produced a valuable concise guide for clinicians on the diagnosis and treatment of various comorbidity conditions when they present with ADHD in children and adolescents.

It is critical to detect, evaluate, and treat comorbid conditions in children and adolescents with ADHD since if this is not done the child or adolescent is not likely to improve in their academic, social, or emotional functioning.

The value and usefulness of this book lies in its various characteristics, namely:

(a) The range of comorbidities it covers;
(b) The language and format used; and
(c) Its extensive referencing.

(a) Range of Comorbidities Covered

The comorbid conditions covered are wide ranging and include anxiety, depression and suicidality, oppositional defiant disorder, conduct disorder, learning disorders, substance abuse disorder, tics disorder and Tourette's syndrome, borderline personality disorder, bipolar disorder, as well as epilepsy and obesity. Some of these comorbidities are common and others are rare. However, most of the common comorbidities have been included.

The wide range of comorbidities covered adds to the value of the book.

(b) Language and Format Used

Language is clear and concise and generally avoids professional jargon, making it comprehensible to most readers, professionals, and laymen alike.

The format used adds to the clarity, conciseness, and usefulness of the book.

Specifically, each chapter starts with a list of objectives which cover the prevalence of the comorbid condition and the challenges in its diagnosis and treatment.

This is followed by a clinical case history which illustrates some of these challenges in diagnoses and treatment.

The chapter proceeds with asking and then answering in point form (with references and tables) key issues pertaining to the prevalence, diagnosis, and treatment of the particular comorbid conditions.

This question and answer format in point or table form with references allows the reader to get key questions answered quickly, concisely, with the option to dive further into the topic by consulting the references.

This format is one of the main strengths of the book.

(c) Extensive Referencing

Each chapter is concluded by an extensive set of references on the topics covered in the chapter, references on prevalence, diagnosis, and treatment. However, references also include assessment instruments, rating scales, as well as treatment resources regarding parenting, family, child, or adolescent treatment studies and interventions.

The references thus constitute a very valuable resource to clinicians and others for further knowledge and tools regarding diagnosis and treatment of the various comorbidities discussed.

In summary, Dr. Sadek has produced a book which will be very valuable to clinicians and laymen alike on a clinically important area, namely the diagnosis and treatment of various comorbid conditions which can accompany ADHD. The detection and treatment of these comorbid conditions is critical for the optimal academic, social, and emotional functioning of children and adolescents with ADHD and thus will be useful to clinicians who treat the patients as well as children, adolescents, and families trying to cope with ADHD and its frequent comorbidities.

Disclaimer

The text in this book and its references are for education, guidance, and information purposes only. Responsibility remains in the hands of the clinician diagnosing and treating their own patient to determine the correct course for their patient. No one who took part in creating this text can be held legally responsible for any of the information contained in the text.

Lily Hechtman
Division of Child Psychiatry
McGill University,
Montreal, QC, Canada

Contents

About the Author and Reviewers

About the Author

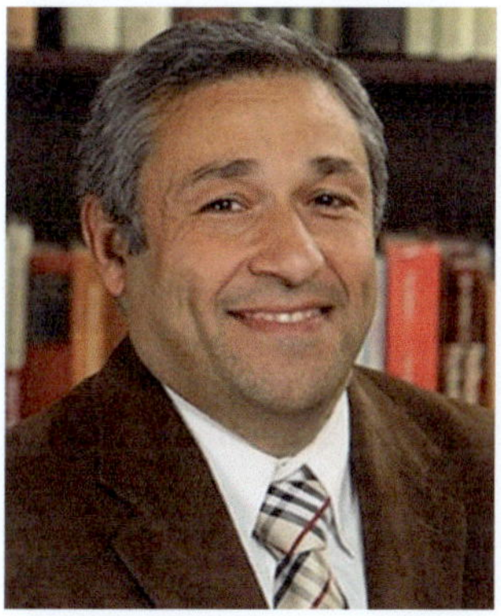

Joseph Sadek is an associate professor of psychiatry at Dalhousie University and the medical director of the Atlantic ADHD Center in Dartmouth, Nova Scotia. He is also the clinical and academic leader, Nova Scotia Hospital, Mayflower Unit, Dartmouth, NS, Canada. Dr. Sadek is a diplomat of the American Board of Psychiatry and Neurology (DABPN) and fellow of the Royal College of Physicians and Surgeons of Canada (FRCPC). In addition to his medical degree (1990), Dr. Sadek also holds a pharmacy degree (B.Sc. Pharm 1986) and an MBA from St. Mary's University. He also completed a one-year research training program at Harvard Medical School and obtained the certification of the Global Clinical Scholars Research Program (GCSRP) with commendation. He completed his psychiatry residency training at Dalhousie University, Nova Scotia, Canada. Dr. Sadek served as the head of the Neurosciences professional competency unit for the Dalhousie Medical School. He started the first public adult ADHD clinic in Nova Scotia in 2007. He is heavily involved in both the undergraduate and postgraduate teaching and has published a book called *Clinician's Guide to ADHD*, second edition, in 2013. A second book called *Clinician's Guide to Adult ADHD Comorbidities* was published in 2016. Dr. Sadek has several peer-reviewed articles and received several quality awards for his work. He served as the vice president of the Canadian ADHD Resource Alliance (CADDRA) and created the CADDRA ADHD Institute in 2012. Dr. Sadek is the chair of the Suicide Prevention Task Force for the Province of Nova Scotia. He was also a member of the Dalhousie University Senate. Dr. Sadek received the Mental Health Program Quality Council Certificate of Excellence Award for commitment to quality review (2012) and Mental Health Program Quality Council Certificate of Excellence Award for development and implementation of suicide risk assessment form (2012). In 2017, he received the Saint Mary's University MBA 25th Anniversary Alumni Impact Award.

About the Reviewers

Alexa Bagnell is an associate professor in the Department of psychiatry, Dalhousie University, and the chief of the IWK Child and Adolescent Psychiatry. She obtained BSc (McGill University), MA (Oxford University), and MD (Dalhousie University). She completed her psychiatry/child residency training at Harvard University. Dr. Bagnell is a clinician researcher and a founder of the Treatment of Anxiety Group (2005) and the OCD Clinic (2013) at the IWK Health Centre. Her research interests are in promoting earlier intervention for mental health disorders, with a focus on schools and web-based programs.

Sue Zinck is an assistant professor of psychiatry at Dalhousie University and a staff psychiatrist at the IWK Health Centre. She received her M.D. from Dalhousie in 1998 and completed both her psychiatry residency in 2004 and fellowship in Child and Adolescent Psychiatry in 2005 at the McGill University Health Centre. Dr. Zinck became a Royal College fellow in Child and Adolescent Psychiatry in 2013, the certification's inaugural year. She is clinical leader at the IWK Bipolar Disorders clinic and with the IWK Transgender Health Team. She is the Psychiatry Co-leader of the IWK Community Mental Health Clinic, Halifax branch.

Normand Carrey is an infant, child, and adolescent psychiatrist-clinician researcher with over 30 years of clinical and research experience. He has been designated as "Founder" for the subspecialty of Child and Adolescent Psychiatry (Royal College of Canada), is the former Editor-in-Chief for the *Journal of the Canadian Academy of Child and Adolescent Psychiatry*, and is currently the Head of Family Therapy, Dalhousie University. He has numerous publications and his main areas of research are (1) realist reviews of parenting interventions for preschoolers within the child welfare system; (2) systemic knowledge mobilization around attachment-based models and interventions for preschoolers (0–5), especially the Circle of Security Intervention (translator of the French version); (3) empathy syndromes (fetal alcohol syndrome, conduct problems—callous-unemotional traits, pervasive developmental disorders), systematic reviews; and (4) models of supervision in family therapy.

Anita Hickey is currently practicing Child and Adolescent Psychiatry at the IWK Health Centre. Her role includes general outpatient psychiatry services, as well as Emergency Department and Consultation Liaison psychiatry coverage. Her research includes oppositional defiant disorder, attachment theory, and 0–5 early year intervention impact on attachment and future behavior. In addition to her psychiatry appointment at the IWK Mental Health and Addictions program, Dr. Hickey is also an assistant professor with the Department of Psychiatry at Dalhousie University.

Lily Hechtman is a professor of psychiatry and pediatrics at McGill University and Director of Research in the Division of Child Psychiatry. She is an internationally recognized researcher and pioneer in ADHD. Part of Dr. Hechtman's research has focused on long-term (15-year) prospective studies of children with ADHD followed into adolescence and adulthood. Dr. Hechtman conducted the first controlled multimodal treatment study on children with ADHD. This study set the stage for the multisite multimodal treatment study (the MTA). She was the head of one of the sites for the MTA. Dr. Hechtman's honors include Children and Adults with Attention Deficit Disorder (CHADD) Hall of Fame (CHADD considers the Hall of Fame to be its highest recognition.); American Academy of Child and Adolescent Psychiatry Elaine Schlosser Lewis Award for research on Attention Deficit Disorder; American Academy of Child and Adolescent Psychiatry Pilot Project Award for Attention Deficit Disorder; Canadian Academy of Child and Adolescent Psychiatry Paul D. Steinhauer Advocacy Award in testament for work as an exceptional advocate for children, adolescents, and their families at the regional, national, and international level; and Canadian Academy of Child and Adolescent Psychiatry Honorary Member Award for an academic career with outstanding contributions in service, teaching, and research at the regional, national, and international level. Dr. Hechtman combines a rigorous research background with extensive clinical expertise and experience.

Introduction

There is a need for a clear and concise approach to a complex disorder such as attention deficit hyperactivity disorder (ADHD). Understanding the diagnosis and management of ADHD is incomplete without understanding comorbidities and how to manage them.

This guide uses a case-based approach to explain several areas in the diagnosis and management of ADHD in the presence of several comorbid disorders in children and adolescents.

Despite the complexity of the topic, each case brings a unique perspective on ADHD patients. The consistent approach in describing the cases allows clinicians to think of a broader differential diagnosis, then come to a clear impression and a management plan.

Each case is supported by a literature review on different areas such as epidemiology, etiology, morbidity, diagnosis, and management.

This book captures some important disorders that co-occur with ADHD such as anxiety disorders, depression, conduct disorder, oppositional defiant disorder, borderline personality disorder in adolescence, obesity, and seizure disorder.

The cases are designed and written to be practical and relevant for clinicians. The literature reviews are extensive and clear.

Several resources are included in this book to help clinicians expand their knowledge on ADHD comorbidities. They include questionnaires, rating scales, web sites, and ample references.

This guide is intended for educational purposes only. There are many areas in the field of ADHD that were not captured in this guide, and readers are encouraged to continue to update their knowledge regularly.

ADHD and Epilepsy

1

1.1 Objectives

- List some of the comorbid psychiatric conditions that are significantly at higher rate in epilepsy than the general population.
- Describe the prevalence rates and some epidemiological data of ADHD in Epilepsy and epilepsy in ADHD.
- List some of the consequences of ADHD symptoms in children with epilepsy
- List some of the challenges of management of ADHD in childhood epilepsy
- Describe some of the treatment considerations when assessing and managing young patients with comorbid ADHD and Epilepsy

1.2 The Case

Read the following case and check if the clinician completed the following tasks in this case?

- Obtained full psychiatric and medical history?
- Used some rating scales or questionnaires during the assessment?
- Obtained collateral history?
- Reviewed functional impairment?
- Conducted appropriate investigations, blood work and physical exam as indicated?
- Documented the assessment?
- Reached a diagnosis and assessed for comorbid disorders?
- Communicated results of the assessment to the patient and family?
- Provided adequate education to patient and family?
- Explained the possible pharmacological and psychosocial treatments and alternatives?
- Provided appropriate management and treatment interventions

J. Sadek, *Clinician's Guide to ADHD Comorbidities in Children and Adolescents*,
https://doi.org/10.1007/978-3-319-45635-5_1

- Explained the risk and benefit of treatment and lack of treatment?
- Referred the patient to other services or resources in the community as indicated?
- Suggested appropriate accommodations?
- Provided a follow up appointment?

1.2.1 Emerson English

Twelve year old boy who is currently in grade 6. He lives with his mother, sister, brother and step father in Nova Scotia. Emerson was diagnosed with ADHD and seizure disorder 5 years ago. His family did not agree to start him on medications for ADHD but he has been on Divalproex sodium 1000 mg at bedtime and his seizure was well controlled.

He had psychoeducational assessment in 2012 that conformed diagnosis of ADHD. His biological father in Ontario.

Family doctor requested a psychiatric consultation due to decline in academic performance and several complaints from teachers that Emerson is not paying attention and very distracted.

His mother and step father came to the interview and reported the following symptoms for more than 50% of the time:

Feeling tired, fatigued, Overeating, Poor ability to think or concentrate
Worried excessively most days about many things
Have unexplained aches and pains
Emerson is not using alcohol or illegal drugs. He has no thoughts to harm himself or others.

In terms of ADHD patient and parents and teacher reports confirmed the following symptoms:

Fails to give close attention to details and making careless mistakes in school
Has difficulty sustaining attention in class and play activities
Does not seem to listen when spoken to directly
Fails to finish school work, chores, or duties regularly
Has difficulty organizing tasks and activities. His room is a complete mess
Avoids, his homework every day and reluctantly engages in tasks requiring sustained mental effort
Loses things necessary for activities (e.g., toys, school assignments, pencils, and books)
Is distracted by extraneous stimuli such as noise or movement.
Is forgetful in daily activities. Mother has to keep reminding him.
Has difficulty awaiting turn
Fidgets with hands and squirms in seat
Has difficulty playing or engaging in leisure activities quietly. He is loud.

Is "on the go" or often acts as if "driven by a motor"
Talks excessively
Blurts out answers before questions have been completed in class and at home.

In terms of ODD parents reported that he does not loses temper and comply.

With adult requests or rules but he often blames others for his mistakes and is often easily annoyed by others.

In terms of Conduct Disorder parents denied all symptoms.

Medical History: No known allergies. Absence seizure diagnosed 5 years ago and has been seizure free for 2 years.

Medication: Divalproex sodium 1000 mg po HS.

Personal and Developmental History:

There were some complications with mother's pregnancy because of hypertension of pregnancy.
The delivery was on time but was caesarean section.
Patient had no gross motor nor fine motor problems or difficulties. Family never noticed any odd behaviour or impairment in social functioning.
Emerson was bullied in grade 3. He is currently in grade 6 and his grades this year had been poor compared to previous years. This year he had one suspension, mathematics problems and need for after school educational support.

Case outcome: Patient's diagnosis with ADHD and seizure disorder was confirmed. A lengthy discussion and education on benefits and risks of treatment with Emerson and his parents took place. The next appointment, a decision was made by everyone to start ADHD treatment due to decline in Emerson's academic achievements. He was started on Methylphenidate CR 20 mg daily and had no new seizures during the 6 month follow up. His academic performance improved and he was also referred to a psychologist to help him with ADHD strategies and techniques to manage his anxiety. Medication was increased to 30 mg orally daily in the morning with no increase in adverse effects.

1.2.2 Questions

What are the comorbid psychiatric conditions that are significantly at higher rate in epilepsy than the general population?

<u>Psychiatric and cognitive</u>

- ADHD (30–40% prevalence)
- Depression
- Anxiety
- Pervasive developmental Disorders
- Psychosis of epilepsy
- Learning Disorders
- Intellectual Disability

- Dementia/ Alzheimer's disease (Seidenberg et al. 2009)

ADHD was reported to be the be the most common disorder in preschoolers and school aged children with epilepsy with equal distribution between boys and girls (Thome-Souza et al. 2004).

The presence of ADHD symptoms at the time of epilepsy onset can be viewed as a major marker of abnormal cognitive development (Hermann et al. 2008)

Describe the epidemiology of epilepsy in patients with ADHD?

The prevalence for epileptiform EEG discharges ranges from 5 to 60% in children with ADHD (Richer et al. 2002).

Population studies suggest that the prevalence of ADHD in childhood epilepsy is between 12 and 17% (Reilly 2011).

One study in a Tertiary Care Centre found that 60% of children with epilepsy met the diagnostic criteria for ADHD. The epilepsy sample observed in that Centre was characterized by early age of onset, significant duration of epilepsy, high seizure frequency, and intractability (Sherman et al. 2007).

Some researchers found more attentional problems in children prior to their first recognized seizure compared with siblings without seizures (Austin et al. 2001). A population-based study in Iceland found a history of ADHD was 2.5 times more likely in new cases of epilepsy than in a control group without epilepsy (Hesdorffer et al. 2004).

Some biological mechanisms have been suggested for the comorbidity of ADHD and epilepsy such as disrupted lipid metabolism, abnormalities in the Norepinephrine (NE) system and dopamine transporter system, increased grey matter frontal lobe volume, decreased brainstem volumes. Psychosocial mechanisms were also suggested (Seidenberg et al. 2009).

List some of the epilepsies associated with ADHD?

- Frontal lobe epilepsy (FLE)
- Childhood absence epilepsy
- Rolandic epilepsy
- Sleep related epilepsies and other subtypes

What are the consequences of ADHD symptoms in children with epilepsy?

- Lower quality of life (Sherman et al. 2007, 2010)
- Academic underperformance (Williams et al. 2001)—Need for more supportive education and formal IEP (Hermann et al. 2007)
- Low achievement scores (scores below age means) for reading, mathematics and writing, but not IQ-achievement (Fastenau et al. 2008)
- Possible increase in anxiety symptoms (Williams et al. 2003)
- Poorer performance in tasks of executive function (Seidenberg et al. 2009)
- In pervasive developmental disorders, some studies suggested that PDD and epilepsy comorbidity is associated with lower IQ, lowered adaptive behaviour scores, more emotional problems, more disruptive behavior and higher psychotropic drug use (Matson and Neal 2009).

What are the principals of assessment of children with Epilepsy and ADHD symptoms?

- Assess for temporal relationships between the course of the epilepsy, and the onset of ADHD
- Assess sleep quality and efficiency and assess for presence of specific sleep disorders
- Obtain a comprehensive neuropsychological evaluation, particularly among children whose academic achievements are deteriorating
- Use EEG monitoring to detect the presence of unrecognized seizures
- Conduct a formal ADHD assessment including child and parents and obtain reports from school

What are the challenges of management of ADHD in childhood epilepsy?

- Lack of robust blind placebo-controlled trials to define the optimal treatment of ADHD symptoms in children with epilepsy (Dunn and Kronenberger 2006),
- Many children with epilepsy may be excluded from the clinical trials or controlled pharmacological studies of medications designed to treat ADHD symptoms (Plioplys et al. 2007).
- Use of generic checklists such as CBCL in children with epilepsy may be misleading due to potential exacerbation of ADHD symptoms by presence of seizure or antiepileptic medications (Reilly 2011)
- Psychostimulant may lower seizure threshold (Gucuyener et al. 2003; Tan and Appleton 2005).
- Methylphenidate (MPH) can increase phenytoin serum concentrations (Markowitz et al. 1999). Furthermore, MPH serum concentrations may be lowered by the administration of carbamazepine, thus leading to a loss of efficacy (Schaller and Behar 1999)

What are the treatment recommendations for ADHD in Childhood epilepsy?

Treatment with psychotropic drugs can be initiated safely in most children with epilepsy and ADHD symptoms (Parisi 2010).

In the UK the National Institute for Health and Clinical Excellence (NICE) clinical guidelines published in 2009 endorse the use of non-pharmacological treatments for children, young people, and adults with ADHD and recommended that pharmacological treatments should always form part of a comprehensive intervention plan that includes psychological, behavioural, and educational advice and interventions (Young and Amarasinghe 2010).

Several researchers advocate that treatment of ADHD in children with epilepsy should be multimodal and it has been proposed that pharmacologic intervention as part of biopsychosocial approach to ADHD can foster learning and good behavioural functioning (Torres et al. 2008; Kaufmann et al. 2009).

Despite the paucity of data, studies suggest that Methylphenidate (MPH) should be considered as a treatment option in children with moderate or severe ADHD and well-controlled seizures.

A meta-analysis concluded that incidence rates of seizures as adverse events were not significantly different between methylphenidate, atomoxetine, and placebo (Wernicke et al. 2007) however one report suggested that atomoxetine induced seizure occurred after overdose (Kashani and Ruha 2007).

Melatonin can be used in sleep disruption in patients with Epilepsy and ADHD.

Clinicians should

1. Optimize seizure control and in the presence of a deterioration in ADHD symptoms. Assess whether a change in epilepsy or ADHD medications is required versus decreasing the number of antiepileptic medications used or switching to an AED with fewer cognitive or behavioral effects
2. Attempt to improve sleep disorders and/or ADHD symptoms by achieving better seizure control
3. Assess periodically for the possibility that ADHD medication is no longer needed.

References

Austin JK, Harezlak J, Dunn DW, Huster GA, Rose DF, Ambrosius WT. Behavior problems in children before first recognized seizures. Pediatrics. 2001;107:115–22.

Dunn DW, Kronenberger WG. Childhood epilepsy, attention problems, and ADHD: review and practical considerations. Semin Pediatr Neurol. 2006;12:222–8.

Fastenau PS, Shen J, Dunn DW, Austin JK. Academic underachievement among children with epilepsy: proportion exceeding psychometric criteria for learning disability and associated risk factors. J Learn Disabil. 2008;41(3):195–207.

Gucuyener K, Erdemoglu K, Senol S, Sedaroglu A, Soysal S, Kockar AI. Use of methylphenidate for attention-deficit hyperactivity disorder in patients with epilepsy or electroencephalographic abnormalities. J Child Neurol. 2003;18:109–12.

Hermann B, Jones J, Dabbs K, Allen CA, Sheth R, Fine J, et al. The frequency, complications and aetiology of ADHD in new onset paediatric epilepsy. Brain. 2007;130:3135–48.

Hermann BP, Jones JE, Sheth R, Koehn M, Becker T, Fine J, et al. Growing up with epilepsy: a two-year investigation of cognitive development in children with new onset epilepsy. Epilepsia. 2008;49:1847–58.

Hesdorffer DC, Ludvigsson P, Olafsson E, Gudmundsson G, Kjartansson O, Hauser WA. ADHD as a risk factor for incident unprovoked seizures and epilepsy in children. Arch Gen Psychiatry. 2004;61:731–6.

Kashani J, Ruha AM. Isolated atomoxetine overdose resulting in seizure. J Emerg Med. 2007;32:175–8.

Kaufmann R, Goldberg-Stern H, Shuper A. Attention-deficit disorders and epilepsy in childhood: incidence, causative relations, and treatment possibilities. J Child Neurol. 2009;24(6):727–33.

Markowitz JS, Morrison SD, DeVane CL. Drug interactions with psychostimulants. Int Clin Psychopharmacol. 1999;14:1–18.

Matson JL, Neal D. Seizures and epilepsy and their relation to autism spectrum disorders. Res Autism Spectr Disord. 2009;3:999–1005.

Plioplys S, Dunn D, Caplan R. 10-year research update review: psychiatric problems in children with epilepsy. J Am Acad Child Adolesc Psychiatry. 2007;46(11):1389–402.

Reilly CJ. Attention deficit hyperactivity disorder (ADHD) in childhood epilepsy. Res Dev Disabil. 2011;32(3):883–93.

Richer LP, Shevell MI, Rosenblatt BR. Epileptiform abnormalities in children with attention-deficit-hyperactivity disorder. Pediatr Neurol. 2002;26:125–9.

Schaller JL, Behar D. Carbamazepine and methylphenidate in ADHD. J Am Acad Child Adolesc Psychiatry. 1999;38:112–3.

Seidenberg M, Pulsipher DT, Hermann B. Association of epilepsy and comorbid conditions. Future Neurol. 2009;4(5):663–8.

Sherman EMS, Slick DJ, Connolly MB, Eyrl KL. ADHD, neurological correlates and health-related quality of life in severe pediatric epilepsy. Epilepsia. 2007;48(6):1083–91.

Sherman EMS, Brooks BL, Akdag S, Connolly MB, Wiebe S. Parents report more ADHD symptoms than do teachers in children with epilepsy. Epilepsy Behav. 2010;19(3):428–35.

Tan M, Appleton R. Attention deficit and hyperactivity disorder, methylphenidate and epilepsy. Arch Dis Child. 2005;90:57–9.

Thome-Souza S, Kuczynski E, Assumpcao F Jr, et al. Which factors may play a pivotal role on determining the type of psychiatric disorder in children and adolescents with epilepsy? Epilepsy Behav. 2004;5:988–94.

Torres AR, Whitney J, Gonzalez-Heydrich J. Attention-deficit hyperactivity disorder in pediatric patients with epilepsy: review of Pharmacological treatment. Epilepsy Behav. 2008;12(2):217–33.

Wernicke JF, Holdridge KC, Jin L, Edison T, Zhang S, Bangs ME, et al. Seizure risk in patients with attention-deficit-hyperactivity disorder treated with atomoxetine. Dev Med Child Neurol. 2007;49:498–502.

Williams J, Schultz EG, Griebel ML. Seizure occurrence in children diagnosed with ADHD. Clin Pediatr. 2001;40:221–4.

Williams J, Steel C, Sharp GB, DelosReyes E, Philips T, Bates S, et al. Anxiety in children with epilepsy. Epilepsy Behav. 2003;4:729–32.

Young S, Amarasinghe M. Practitioner review: non-pharmacological treatments for ADHD: a lifespan approach. J Child Psychol Psychiatry. 2010;51(2):116–33.

2 ADHD and Borderline Personality Disorder (BPD) in Adolescence

2.1 Objectives

- Review the epidemiology and etiology of ADHD and BPD
- Describe the challenges around the diagnosis of Borderline Personality Disorder (BPD) in Adolescents
- list some of the warning signs that may point to presence of BPD in adolescence
- Recognize the importance of identifying comorbid personality disorder in patients with ADHD
- Understand the management approaches for patients with BPD and ADHD
- Recognize the challenges in treatment of ADHD in presence of BPD.

2.2 The Case

Read the following case and check if the clinician completed the following tasks in this case?

- Obtained full psychiatric and medical history?
- Used some rating scales or questionnaires during the assessment?
- Obtained collateral history?
- Reviewed functional impairment?
- Conducted appropriate investigations, blood work and physical exam as indicated?
- Documented the assessment?
- Reached a diagnosis and assessed for comorbid disorders?
- Communicated results of the assessment to the patient and family?
- Provided adequate education to patient and family?
- Explained the possible pharmacological and psychosocial treatments and alternatives?

J. Sadek, *Clinician's Guide to ADHD Comorbidities in Children and Adolescents*,
https://doi.org/10.1007/978-3-319-45635-5_2

- Provided appropriate management and treatment interventions
- Explained the risk and benefit of treatment and lack of treatment?
- Referred the patient to other services or resources in the community as indicated?
- Suggested appropriate accommodations?
- Provided a follow up appointment?

2.3 Barbara B

- BB is a healthy 17 year old single female who lives alone in Portland, Main. She is currently in grade 12.
- Patient was brought to her family doctor by her mother after BB told her mother that she has been cutting her arms when her boyfriend decided to leave her. They were together for 1 month.

2.3.1 History of Present Illness and Review of Systems

- Barbara has been very upset the past week because her new boyfriend left her. They were dating for 1 month then he told her that he does not wish to continue this relationship.
- Mood symptoms: patient reported hourly mood changes that range from irritability to depression or sudden happiness. She also reported lack of motivation and procrastinating. She has been trying to lose weight, despite having ideal body weight. Barbara watches what she eats but does not restrict her food intake. Once a week, she may binge and purge. 2 years ago, she was a teenager she used several laxatives but she does not use them anymore. She describes 4 years of feelings of low self-esteem but her energy and appetite are good. She enjoys outdoor activities, watching movies, and playing video games. She has no suicidal intent or plans but she threatens suicide if she does not get what she wants. When stressed she scratches her arm. Her attention and concentrate have been described as poor as long as she remembers. Denies feelings of guilt and her sleep is poor with frequent awakening in the middle of the night. She thinks that most of her symptoms started when she was 13 years old.
- Anxiety symptoms: Patient has chronic worry about people not liking her and not being the center of attention despite her appearance and ideal body weight. She can control her worries but feels restless all the time. Negative screening for phobia, Obsessive compulsive disorder (OCD), panic disorder.
- Alcohol and substance use: Barbara will binge drink weekly and on weekends she drinks 12–24 beers until she is drunk. She is open to trying street drugs when offered in parties. She used Cocaine and LSD 2 years ago but did not use them since. Currently she uses small amounts of weed when she cannot sleep. She started drinking and using drugs at age 14. She does not see alcohol use as a problem. She describes it as helpful and fun.
- Psychosis: Barbara feels that people talk about her behind her back. “They do not like me and stare at me” she said and she stopped interacting with many of them. Screening for hallucinations and delusions was negative.

- **Past psychiatric history:** Multiple short admissions (less than 4 days) to hospital over the past 3 years. She was referred for outpatient mental health but she never showed up. She has been on Fluoxetine, which she stopped after few weeks because of intolerable nausea and refused to try any mother medication.
- **Medical history:** No known allergy. Healthy. Had one abortion at age 15.
- **Family History**: Barbara has one sister. Parents divorced when she was 4 years old. Barbara's paternal grandparents abused drugs and alcohol. Her mother and sister have been diagnosed with depression and anxiety. Her sister also suffers from ADHD.
- **Developmental, Personal and social History**: Her mother smoked cigarettes while pregnant with BB, but consumed neither street drugs nor alcohol. The delivery was vaginal and patient had no delay in developmental milestones. She was described as hyperactive child who was accident prone. During elementary school she received average marks and was often defiant with teachers. Teachers frequently commented that she does not finish her homework. She does not listen in class and talks too much and distracts other kids. She hated school but was able to get along well with other children. She failed grade 6 after a year of sexual abuse by her step-father. Her mother found out and left him. BB feels that she never received affection and love as a child. School performance improved slightly in high school after having a very supportive guidance counsellor. She had difficulty paying attention in class and found mathematics very challenging that she always needed tutoring and extra support. Her report cards mentioned consistently that she cannot pay attention in class and that she is easily distracted. BB said that she has difficulty sitting down to do her homework and she cannot finish reading more than few pages of any book that she starts. She describes significant difficulties sustaining her attention in class. Her mind always wonders. Her room is very messy and disorganized. She avoided the assignments in school because it requires focusing and paying attention, but her mother had to force her to sit down and complete her work.
- On the positive note, BB is very artistic and has won a number of awards for her paintings and dance performances. Socially, she has two close friends, although she says, "some days I feel they hate me but I do not want them to leave me. They do not like that I interrupt them all the time but I do not care."

2.3.1.1 Collateral History

Patient consented to talking to her mother Linda who confirmed the following.

Mother had to force Barbara to sit down and complete her homework because she avoids doing it. Barbara lost so many items during elementary school and her mother had to go to school frequently to try to find them. These items included her jacket, her gym shirts, her books and her homework. Barbara was described as "easily distracted and very disorganized". Her room is very messy. She was very talkative and loud but now she does not talk nearly as much. Brenda does not listen because of day dreaming all the time.

She has severe mood swings and could destroy the furniture when she is angry. Barbara binge drinks and can be very impulsive in spending the money she gets and keeps going to her mother to borrow money. Mom is very concerned about her promiscuous behavior, heavy drinking and the self-harm.

At this point Brenda was referred to see a psychiatrist.

2.3.2 Summary of the Findings and Management of This Patient

After reviewing the collateral history, interviewing the patient and completing the assessment, the psychiatrist listed the following disorders in the initial diagnostic impression:

ADHD inattentive type, Alcohol use disorder, Borderline personality disorder and history of eating disorder NOS.

The psychiatrist

- Ordered blood work including TSH that all appeared within normal limits,
- Asked the patient and mother and teachers to complete several rating scales and questionnaires.
- Explained his diagnostic impression to Barbara including all the symptoms of Borderline Personality disorder.
- Provided her with education and useful books and websites including www.DBTselfhelp.com. Barbara was delighted to understand her symptoms and was relieved to hear that her problems are not diagnosed as depression since she tried so many antidepressants in the past with no success.
- Referred her to dialectical behavioural therapy for adolescence (DBT-A). She agreed to start DBT-A psychotherapy program
- Measured her blood pressure, pulse, weight and height. Her blood pressure was 110/76 and pulse was 81. Weight was 140 lbs and height 5′9"
- Started her on a stimulant medication (Lisdexamfetamine 20 mg) in the morning.
- Prescribed melatonin 5 mg at bedtime that improved her sleep.
- Described to her the benefits and risk of medications and she felt agreed to start the treatment.
- Referred her back to her family doctor after starting the DBT-A program and tolerating the medication well (2 follow up visits). She was able to continue to go to school and started working in a grocery store. 6 month after starting treatment for ADHD and BPD, her symptoms were much improved.

2.4 Literature Review Questions

2.4.1 Discuss the Challenges Around the Diagnosis of Borderline Personality Disorder (BPD) in Adolescents?

Clinicians in several parts of the world are reluctant to diagnose BPD in adolescents for the following reasons:

1. The diagnosis of BPD may be invalid in adolescence.
2. Common features of BPD, such as affective instability or disturbed self-image, are normative among adolescents.

3. Personality could still be in development.
4. BPD diagnosis can be stigmatizing and clinicians wish to protect their patients from stigmatizing and pessimistic attitudes.

Recently, a review concluded that research did not support the first 3 assumptions and lots of work is being done to change the stigma associated with BPD. BPD has been found to be a reliable and valid diagnosis in adolescence. Early intervention is beneficial (Kaess et al. 2016).

2.4.2 Discuss the Epidemiology and Comorbidity of ADHD and Borderline Personality Disorder (BPD)?

Attention deficit/hyperactivity disorder (ADHD) is seen as a neuro-developmental disorder starting before the age of 12, according to the DSM-V. More than 50% of the children suffering from ADHD still displayed clinically relevant symptoms when reaching adulthood, with a high degree of psychiatric comorbidities (Kessler et al. 2006), among which borderline personality disorder (BPD) is encountered more often than expected by chance. (Bernardi et al. 2012; Philipsen et al. 2008).

ADHD is characterized by a persistent pattern of inattention and/or hyperactivity/impulsivity that can interfere with or reduce the quality of social, academic or occupational functioning. However, when diagnosing ADHD in adults, it is important to note that the expression of key symptoms can change with age. In particular, hyperactivity and impulsiveness tend to decline with increasing age, whereas inattention tends to persist (Biederman et al. 2000; Larsson et al. 2011). Symptoms such as hyperactivity may change into feelings of inner tension or restlessness (Kooij et al. 2010), which can then be mistaken as signs of anxiety or depression.

In some cases, the diagnosis of ADHD can be difficult, particularly when the disorder is severe and presents with mental health symptoms that may mimic those of other mental health disorders such as borderline personality disorder (BPD) (Perugi et al. 2012; Van Dijk et al. 2012). At times, symptoms that overlap with those of ADHD and can lead to inaccurate diagnosis, and or management.

Failure to recognize a comorbid personality disorder in patients with ADHD may lead to the wrong assumption of treatment failure if pharmacotherapy for ADHD does not bring about adequate clinical and functional improvement. In addition, individuals with ADHD and comorbid borderline personality disorder may need additional interventions, such as dialectical behavioral therapy, to address serious symptoms such as self-injury and distorted perception (Lieb et al. 2004, 2010).

In adolescence, Point prevalence estimate of BPD is around 0.9%. Cumulative prevalence rates suggest that 1.4% of adolescents will meet diagnostic criteria for BPD by age 16 years, and 3.2% by age 22 years. The diagnostic stability of BPD has been found to be similar in adolescents and adults (Kaess et al. 2016).

Comorbidity rates between ADHD and Borderline personality disorder (BPD) are well documented in the literature. The overlap may seem unusually strong. For example, Philipsen et al. (2008) found only 16% comorbidity of BPD with ADHD. On the other hand, a more recent study (Ferrer et al. 2010) reported a number as high as 38%.

Both ADHD and Borderline personality disorder have indistinguishable comorbidity rates for substance use, anxiety and eating disorders, and very similar levels of cyclothymia, which may point to mood labiality as a common denominator of these disorders (Perugi et al. 2012).

2.4.3 List Some of the Different Hypothesis That Are Proposed to Account for the Comorbidity Between ADHD and BPD?

1. The comorbid disorders do not represent distinct entities but, rather are the expression phenotypic variability of the same disorder.
2. Each of the comorbid disorders represents distinct and separate clinical entities.
3. The comorbid disorders share common vulnerabilities, either genetic (genotype), psychosocial (adversity), or both.
4. The comorbid disorders represent a distinct subtype (genetic variant) within a heterogeneous disorder.
5. One syndrome is an early manifestation of the comorbid disorder (i.e. ADHD is an early manifestation of a mood disorder).
6. The development of one syndrome increases the risk for the comorbid disorder (i.e. ADHD increases the risk for borderline personality disorder). Investigations of these issues should help to clarify the etiology, course, and outcome of ADHD (Davids and Gastpar 2005).

2.4.4 What Are the Diagnostic Symptoms Criteria of Borderline Personality Disorder?

According to DSM V (APA 2013), patient has to have a long standing pattern that started in early adulthood that causes significant impairment in function and meets 5 of the following criteria:

- An intense fear of abandonment, even going to extreme measures to avoid real or imagined rejection or abandonment
- A pattern of unstable intense relationships, sometimes seeing things as black and white or using splitting as a defense
- Rapid changes in self-identity or self-image that include shifting goals and values.
- Periods of stress-related paranoia and loss of contact with reality, lasting from a few minutes to a few hours.
- Impulsive and risky behavior, such as, reckless driving, sex, spending sprees, binge eating or drug abuse or gambling.
- Suicidal threats or behavior or self-injury, often in response to fear of separation or rejection.
- Significant and wide mood changes or swings that can happen within the same day, lasting from a few hours to a few days, which can include intense happiness, irritability, or anxiety.

- Long standing feelings of emptiness
- Inappropriate, severe anger episodes or difficulty controlling anger, such as frequently losing temper, being sarcastic or bitter, or having physical fights

2.4.5 What Are Some of the Warning Signs That May Point to Presence of BPD in Adolescence?

Repetitive non suicidal self-injury (NSSI) or suicide attempts
Impulsive risk-taking behaviors (e. g, substance abuse, risky sexual behavior)
Mixture of high levels of both internalizing (depressive symptoms, anxiety) and externalizing problems (conduct problems)
Frequent anger outbursts
Frequent interpersonal problems and unstable relationships
Insecure identity, lack of goals in life and very low self-esteem (Kaess et al. 2016)

2.4.6 Describe Some of the Key Similarities and Differences Between Borderline Personality Disorder and ADHD?

Both disorders are chronic, disabling and impairing conditions that are pervasive across many situations and might share impulsivity as a common symptom (ADHD combined type and Hyperactive-impulsive type). ADHD has childhood onset or early adolescent onset while BPD has Early adult/adolescent onset; signs in childhood in some cases. Some key differences: Inattention is not a core feature of BPD however frantic efforts to avoid real or imagined abandonment is one of the core feature of BPD. Recurrent suicidal behaviour is a core feature of BPD but not ADHD. Hourly mood fluctuation is a core feature of BPD but some affective lability might be found in ADHD (Asherson et al. 2014).

Some neuroimaging studies suggest that for ADHD and BPD, there may be some shared neurobiological dysfunction, thus a degree of overlap may exist in underlying brain dysfunctions, as well as in symptomatology. For instance, there may be dysfunctions of the prefrontal cortex, a core region for attentional mechanisms and impulse control, and in the orbitofrontal cortex, a core region for impulsivity and emotional control (Broome et al. 2015).

Anger expression and aggression are reported to be higher in comorbid BPD and ADHD (Prada et al. 2014).

2.4.7 What Are the Management Difficulties in Patients with Comorbid ADHD and BPD That Are Related to BPD?

Patients with BPD can be difficult to manage for a number of reasons. For one they often elicit countertransference reactions in the treating physician which can lead to the over or under prescription of pharmaceuticals. Patients with BPD may struggle with accurately assessing response to ADHD medications. As such it is important to rely on objective measures when gauging response to treatment. It is also very important to maintain appropriate boundaries at all times with BPD patients. When patient expectations are not met, they may react with feelings of abandonment, rage, disappointment, or devaluation (Gabbard and Wilkinson 2000).

2.4.8 Why Is It Important to Recognize a Comorbid Personality Disorder in Patients with ADHD?

Failure to recognize a comorbid personality disorder in patients with ADHD may lead to the wrong assumption of treatment failure if pharmacotherapy for ADHD does not lead to adequate clinical and functional improvement.

In addition, individuals with ADHD and comorbid borderline personality disorder may need additional interventions, such as dialectical behavioral therapy, to address serious symptoms such as self-injury and distorted perception (Lieb et al. 2004; Mao and Findling 2014).

2.4.9 What Are the Potential Advantages of a Dimensional Model over a Categorical Model in Diagnosing BPD?

When a dimensional approach is used, sub-threshold conditions can be easily identified and described and changes in symptoms over time can be more detected. In addition, therapeutic interventions could be more individually targeted (Schmeck et al. 2013; Widiger and Simonsen 2005).

2.4.10 What Are Some of the Helpful Tips for Managing Borderline Patients in Primary Care Setting?

- Learn about common clinical presentations and causes of undesirable behavior.
- Validate the patient's feelings by naming the emotion you suspect, such as fear of abandonment, anger, shame, and so on, before addressing the "facts" of the situation and acknowledge the real stresses in the patient's situation.
- Avoid responding to provocative behavior.
- Schedule regular, time-limited visits that are not contingent on the patient being "sick."
- Set clear boundaries at the beginning of the treatment relationship and do not respond to attempts to operate outside of these boundaries unless it is a true emergency.
- Make open communication with all other providers a condition of treatment.
- Avoid polypharmacy and large-volume prescriptions of potentially toxic medications (including tricyclic antidepressants, cardiac medications, and benzodiazepines).
- Avoid prescribing potentially addicting medications such as benzodiazepines or opiates. Inform patients of your policies regarding these medications early in the treatment relationship so they are aware of your limits.

- Set firm limits on manipulative behavior while avoiding being judgmental.
- Do not reward difficult behavior with more contact and attention. Provide attention based on a regular schedule rather than being contingent on behavior (Dubovsky and Kiefer 2014).

2.4.11 What Are the Key Clinical Treatment Recommendations in Patients with BPD and ADHD?

Psychotherapy is the primary treatment for BPD. Principals of Dialectic behavior therapy (DBT) may be helpful in ADHD patients as an adjunct to medications.

No fully evidence-based pharmacotherapy exists for the core BPD symptoms although some medications may be effective for individual symptom domains. E.g. impulsivity.

Treatment of ADHD should be considered when treating comorbid personality disorders. Treating the core syndrome of ADHD may result in better functioning, less distress, more control over behavior and possibly will have more engagement and benefit from psychotherapy (Asherson et al. 2014; Philipsen 2006).

2.4.12 Give Examples of Psychotherapeutic Approaches for Patients with BPD?

Examples of empirically studied treatments for BPD include: Dialectic behavior therapy (DBT), mentalization-based therapy, transference-focused psychotherapy, and general psychiatric management.

Several types of these psychotherapies have a manual and require therapists to undergo extensive training, to be self-aware and have access to therapy or consultation by other colleagues to avoid burnout.

DBT is one of the most commonly used approaches for the psychotherapeutic treatment of adolescent BPD. It is an outpatient based treatment involving group and individual therapy and considered as an effctive treatment for BPD. DBT adolescents (DBT-A) consists of 20 weekly individual psychotherapy sessions, weekly participation in the skills group and rigorous supervision of the therapists. The integration of families is a central component of DBT-A.

DBT focuses on teaching the patient how to regulate emotions, manage self-destructive feelings and behaviors, tolerate distress, and develop interpersonal effectiveness and ability to reality testing. It uses different techniques over at least 1 year, including acceptance, and mindfulness. It has been found to reduce self-harm and suicidality in addition to lowering health care costs and utilization of emergency department and inpatient admission (Rathus and Miller 2002).

Mentalization-based therapy is another group and individual psychotherapy. The goal of treatment is focused on helping the patient to “mentalize” or understand the mental state of oneself and others and to think before reacting. It uses psychodynamic approach and is linked to attachment theory (Chanen and McCutcheon 2013).

Transference-focused psychotherapy is an individual, twice-weekly therapy derived from psychoanalysis. It is focused on transference (feelings of the patient projected onto the therapist), and is among the more difficult techniques to learn. It has been developed by Kernberg and his group in accordance with object relations theory. It combines classic analytic techniques with a more structured and presence-focused approach that fits the needs of adolescents with BPD (Foelsch et al. 2008).

General psychiatric management is a once-weekly psychodynamic therapy. It focuses on the patient's interpersonal relationships and can also include pharmacotherapy and family therapy. This is the most available and easiest to learn. In general, effective treatment requires the patient's active involvement and commitment (Dubovsky and Kiefer 2014).

Cognitive analytic therapy (CAT) is used in adolescent BPD and has been adapted for early intervention. CAT is a time-limited, integrative psychotherapy that arose from a theoretical and practical integration of elements of psychoanalytic object relations theory and cognitive psychology, subsequently developing into an integrated model of development and psychopathology.

CAT uses collaboration between patient and therapist where they both reach a shared understanding of the origin of patient's problems, feelings, behaviors and interpersonal relationship difficulties (Chanen et al. 2009).

Other examples include cognitive behavioural therapy (CBT), dynamic deconstructive psychotherapy (DDP), and interpersonal therapy for BPD (IPT-BPD) (Stoffers et al. 2012).

2.4.13 Is There Any Evidence for Mindfulness Based Interventions in ADHD and BPD?

Although only few studies have investigated the effectiveness of mindfulness training in ADHD (many of which showing methodological limitations), some researchers do suggest that mindfulness may be useful in ADHD interventions. Mindfulness means paying attention and being aware of the experiences occurring in the present moment, and some authors argue that mindfulness training is associated with improved attention systems and self-regulation, and that it therefore fosters those skills that are underdeveloped in individuals with ADHD (Schmiedeler 2015).

2.4.14 What Is the General Approach to Pharmacotherapy for BPD?

Cochrane review of 27 trials stated that the current evidence from randomised controlled trials suggests that drug treatment, especially with mood stabilisers and second-generation antipsychotics, may be effective for treating a number of core symptoms and associated psychopathology, but the evidence does not currently support effectiveness for overall severity of borderline personality disorder. Pharmacotherapy should therefore be targeted at specific symptoms (Lieb et al. 2010).

In adolescence, the risks of polypharmacy and iatrogenic harm are high.

One study shows some preliminary evidence for Omega-3-fatty acids in adolescents with BPD and psychosis but no studies in BPD and ADHD.

2.4.15 What Are the Literature Recommendations for Pharmacological Therapy for Patients with ADHD and BPD?

There appears to be very limited data in relation to treatment of patients with comorbid ADHD-BPD (Prada et al. 2015).

Some reviewers argued that, while many patients with BPD receive 'off label' medications, no robust evidence of efficacy exists for pharmacotherapies in relation to "the core BPD symptoms of chronic feelings of emptiness, identity disturbance and abandonment".

Patients with BPD may have some tendencies to misuse or abuse controlled substances therefore careful prescribing should take place particularly for short acting stimulant medications (Stoffers and Lieb 2015).

With regard to the noradrenergic systems, clonidine treatment, which has been reported to effectively reduce impulsivity and hyperactivity in children and adolescents with ADHD, may also reduce aversive inner tension and the urge to self-harm in patients with BPD (Philipsen et al. 2004).

One author suggests that treating the core syndrome of ADHD may result in better functioning, less distress and more control over behavior and possibly will have more engagement and benefit from psychotherapy (Asherson et al. 2014).

References

American Psychiatric Association. Diagnostic and statistical manual of mental disorders, fifth edition (DSM-5). Arlington, VA: American Psychiatric Publishing; 2013.

Asherson P, Young AH, Eich-Höchli D, Moran P, Porsdal V, Deberdt W. Differential diagnosis, comorbidity, and treatment of attention-deficit/hyperactivity disorder in relation to bipolar disorder or borderline personality disorder in adults. Curr Med Res Opin. 2014;30(8):1657–72.

Bernardi S, Faraone SV, Cortese S, Kerridge BT, Pallanti S, Wang S, Blanco C. The lifetime impact of attention deficit hyperactivity disorder: results from the National Epidemiologic Survey on alcohol and related conditions (NESARC). Psychol Med. 2012;42:875–87.

Biederman J, Mick E, Faraone SV. Age-dependent decline of symptoms of attention deficit hyperactivity disorder: impact of remission definition and symptom type. Am J Psychiatry. 2000;157:816–8.

Broome MR, He Z, Iftikhar M, Eyden J, Marwaha S. Neurobiological and behavioural studies of affective instability in clinical populations: a systematic review. Neurosci Biobehav Rev. 2015;51:243–54.

Chanen AM, McCutcheon L. Prevention and early intervention for borderline personality disorder: current status and recent evidence. Br J Psychiatry Suppl. 2013;54:s24–9.

Chanen AM, McCutcheon LK, Germano D, Nistico H, Jackson HJ, McGorry PD. The HYPE clinic: an early intervention service for borderline personality disorder. J Psychiatr Pract. 2009;15(3):163–72.

Davids E, Gastpar M. Attention deficit hyperactivity disorder and borderline personality disorder. Prog Neuropsychopharmacol Biol Psychiatry. 2005;29(6):865–77.

Dubovsky AN, Kiefer MM. Borderline personality disorder in the primary care setting. Med Clin North Am. 2014;98(5):1049–64.
Ferrer M, Andión O, Matalí J, Valero S, Navarro JA, Ramos-Quiroga JA, et al. Comorbid ADHD in borderline patients defines an impulsive subtype of borderline personality disorder. J Personal Disord. 2010;24:812–22.
Foelsch PA, Odom AE, Kernberg OF. Treatment of adolescents with identity diffusion: a modification of transference focused psychotherapy [in French]. Sante Ment Que. 2008;33(1):37–60.
Gabbard G, Wilkinson S. Management of countertransference with borderline patients. Northvale, NJ: Jason Aronson, Inc; 2000. ISBN-10: 0765702630.
Kaess M, Brunner R, Parzer P, Edanackaparampil M, Schmidt J, Kirisgil M, Fischer G, Wewetzer C, Lehmkuhl G, Resch F. Association of adolescent dimensional borderline personality pathology with past and current nonsuicidal self-injury and lifetime suicidal behavior: a clinical multicenter study. Psychopathology. 2016;49(5):356–63.
Kessler RC, Adler L, Barkley R, Biederman J, Conners CK, et al. The prevalence and correlates of adult ADHD in the United States: results from the National Comorbidity Survey Replication. Am J Psychiatr. 2006;163:716–23.
Kooij SJ, Bejerot S, Blackwell A, et al. European consensus statement on diagnosis and treatment of adult ADHD: the European Network Adult ADHD. BMC Psychiatry. 2010;10:67.
Larsson H, Dilshad R, Lichtenstein P, et al. Developmental trajectories of DSM-IV symptoms of attention-deficit/hyperactivity disorder: genetic effects, family risk and associated psychopathology. J Child Psychol Psychiatry. 2011;52:954–63.
Lieb K, Zanarini MC, Schmahl C, Linehan MM, Bohus M. Borderline personality disorder. Lancet. 2004;364(9432):453–61.
Lieb K, Völlm B, Rücker G, Timmer A, Stoffers JM. Pharmacotherapy for borderline personality disorder: Cochrane systematic review of randomised trials. Br J Psychiatry. 2010;196(1):4–12.
Mao AR, Findling RL. Comorbidities in adult attention-deficit/hyperactivity disorder: a practical guide to diagnosis in primary care. Postgrad Med. 2014;126(5):42–51.
Perugi G, Toni C, Maremmani I, Tusini G, Ramacciotti S, et al. The influence of affective temperaments and psychopathological traits on the definition of bipolar disorder subtypes: a study on bipolar I Italian national sample. J Affect Disord. 2012;136:e41–9.
Philipsen A. Differential diagnosis and comorbidity of attention-deficit/hyperactivity disorder (ADHD) and borderline personality disorder (BPD) in adults. Eur Arch Psychiatry Clin Neurosci. 2006;256(Suppl 1):i42–6.
Philipsen A, Richter H, Schmahl C, Peters J, Rüsch N, Bohus M, Lieb K. Clonidine in acute aversive inner tension and self-injurious behavior in female patients with borderline personality disorder. J Clin Psychiatry. 2004;65(10):1414–9.
Philipsen A, Limberger MF, Lieb K, Feige B, Kleindienst N, Ebner-Priemer U, Barth J, Schmahl C, Bohus M. Attention-deficit hyperactivitydisorder as apotentiallyaggravatingfactorinborderlinepersonalitydisorder. Br J Psychiatr. 2008;192:118–23.
Prada P, Hasler R, Baud P, Bednarz G, Ardu S, Krejci I, Nicastro R, Aubry JM, Perroud N. Distinguishing borderline personality disorder from adult attention deficit/hyperactivity disorder: a clinical and dimensional perspective. Psychiatry Res. 2014;217(1–2):107–14.
Prada P, Nicastro R, Zimmermann J, Hasler R, Aubry JM, Perroud N. Addition of methylphenidate to intensive dialectical behaviour therapy for patients suffering from comorbid borderline personality disorder and ADHD: a naturalistic study. Atten Defic Hyperact Disord. 2015;7(3):199–209.
Rathus JH, Miller AL. Dialectical behavior therapy adapted for suicidal adolescents. Suicide Life Threat Behav. 2002;32(2):146–57.
Schmeck K, Schlüter-Müller S, Foelsch PA, Doering S. The role of identity in the DSM-5 classification of personality disorders. Child Adolesc Psychiatry Ment Health. 2013;7(1):27.
Schmiedeler S. Mindfulness-based intervention in ADHD. Z Kinder Jugendpsychiatr Psychother. 2015;43(2):123–31.
Stoffers JM, Völlm BA, Rücker G, Timmer A, Huband N, Lieb K. Psychological therapies for people with borderline personality disorder. Cochrane Database Syst Rev. 2012;8:CD005652.

Stoffers JM, Lieb K. Pharmacotherapy for borderline personality disorder–current evidence and recent trends. Curr Psychiatry Rep. 2015;17(1):534.
Van Dijk FE, Lappenschaar M, Kan CC, Buitelaar JK, et al. Symptomatic overlap between attention-deficit/hyperactivity disorder and borderline personality disorder in women: the role of temperament and character traits. Compr Psychiatry. 2012;53(1):39–47.
Widiger TA, Simonsen E. Alternative dimensional models of personality disorder: finding a common ground. J Personal Disord. 2005;19(2):110–30.

ADHD and Anxiety

3

3.1 Objectives

- Describe the prevalence rates and some epidemiological data of ADHD and anxiety
- List the overlapping and differentiating symptoms between ADHD and Anxiety disorders
- Describe some of the difficulties in conducting meta-analysis on the effect of stimulant medications on comorbid anxiety in ADHD patients in the current literature
- List some of the instruments that would assist clinicians in identifying different anxiety disorders
- Describe some of the treatment considerations when managing comorbid ADHD and anxiety disorders

3.2 The Case

3.2.1 Amanda Austin

11 year old girl in grade 6 who came to see her new family doctor with her parents because of recent school reports suggestive that Amanda's school performance has been deteriorating.

Father is an accountant and mother is a lawyer.

3.2.2 History of Present Illness

Parents reported a long history of school difficulties. Amanda had to repeat grade 1 because of lack of attendance. In her first few years of school, she would cry each morning when leaving home, cling to her mother and demand to stay home. When

J. Sadek, *Clinician's Guide to ADHD Comorbidities in Children and Adolescents*,
https://doi.org/10.1007/978-3-319-45635-5_3

her father is late, she becomes very anxious and wonders if something bad has happened to him. She has difficulty sleeping because she cannot stop worrying about the health of her parents. She cannot sleep because of her racing thoughts. Amanda always had difficulty finishing her homework. She needed extra help after school and her mother had to sit with her for long periods to help with her homework. Amanda has been constantly losing things in school such as her books and notes. She does not interrupt others or talk over them, and is quite shy and introverted. Her parents also mentioned that she gets bored easily and has difficulty staying focused for more than a few minutes. She is easily distracted particularly with noise or someone moving around.

Parents are also concerned about her trouble staying motivated, irritable mood, constant fidgeting, restlessness and forgetfulness in everyday activities. Teachers had very similar concerns particularly around inattention in classroom, failure to complete her homework, constant need for reassurance, and frequent absenteeism because Amanda feels too tired in the mornings to go.

Amanda never had any therapy and does not take any medications.

3.2.2.1 Medical History

Amanda has no known drug allergies. She had no history of serious medical problems, surgeries or hospitalizations.

No history of any major childhood illnesses and she received all her vaccinations appropriately in a timely fashion. Blood work did not reveal any abnormal findings. She reports stomach upset and nausea when teachers demand that she stays after school to finish her homework.

3.2.2.2 Family History

Amanda's mother has been diagnosed with generalized anxiety disorder and has been stable on Fluoxetine 20 mg daily for 7 years. Father had struggled with alcohol abuse about 8 years ago but has been sober for 2 years. Her older sister Sarah has been diagnosed with ADHD combined type at age 6 and has been stable on Vyvanse (Lisdexamfetamine) 30 mg in the morning for 2 years.

3.2.2.3 Personal and Developmental History

Amanda was the product of an uncomplicated pregnancy. She was born in Halifax, Nova Scotia. Delivery was on time and was a vaginal delivery.

Her developmental motor and language milestones were met in a timely manner.

She was born in intact family and has one older sister (15). She enjoys close relationship with her mother but does not feel as close to her father whom she reports works long hours. She denies any exposure to physical, sexual, or emotional abuse or domestic violence. There is no history of significant loss or negative life events.

Amanda has 2 close friends that she has had since grade 1.

She enjoys playing soccer and loves to play piano.

3.2.2.4 Case Outcome

Patient was diagnosed with ADHD inattentive type and Generalized Anxiety Disorder (GAD). She responded well to cognitive behavioural therapy (CBT) and OROS Methylphenidate 18 mg daily in the morning.

Her blood pressure remained stable at 100/65 and pulse is 71. Height and weight were also monitored.

3.3 Literature Review Questions on ADHD and Anxiety

3.3.1 Describe the Prevalence Rates and Epidemiological Data of ADHD and Anxiety?

The MTA Cooperative Group suggested that the comorbidity rates of ADHD and anxiety in children and adolescents is 33.5% in clinical presentations (The MTA Cooperative Group 1999). The comorbidity rates of ADHD and anxiety in adults have been estimated to be up to 50% (Kessler et al. 2006). In a longitudinal study, patients with ADHD have developed anxiety disorders more frequently than those without ADHD (17.7% vs. 1.9%) and also at an earlier age than the healthy control group (Tai et al. 2013).

- Most common anxiety disorders are simple phobias or separation anxiety in early childhood; social anxiety and generalized anxiety becomes more prevalent with age.
- Risk of anxiety is associated with: earlier inattention moreso than impulsive-hyperactive symptoms (Reinke and Ostrander 2008), greater disruptive and stressful life events, presence of autistic spectrum disorders, chronic multiple tics and parental anxiety disorders.
- Comorbid cases often show lower levels of impulsiveness and they have more sleep problems (bedtime resistance and night waking) but are still more impaired than ADHD only cases.
- Anxiety and ADHD both contribute to social impairment and challenges (Gadow et al. 2009).

3.3.2 What Are the Overlapping and Differentiating Symptoms Between ADHD and Anxiety?

	Overlapping symptoms	Differentiating symptoms
GAD	Difficulty concentrating and distractibility >6 months Restlessness Onset of symptoms are common in childhood	Excessive anxiety and worries that the patient finds difficult to control and is associated with symptoms such as easily fatigued, muscle tension, irritability and sleep disturbance

	Overlapping symptoms	Differentiating symptoms
Panic disorder	Decrease concentration and attention Cause significant distress or impairment in social, academic, occupational or any important area of functioning	Presence of recurrent panic attacks with physical symptoms such as palpitations, sweating, trembling, chills or cognitive symptoms Worry about having additional panic attacks
Agoraphobia	Decrease concentration and significant distress or impairment in social, academic, occupational or any important area of functioning	Fear or anxiety of being in public places, enclosed places, using public transportation, standing in line or with a crowd or leaving home alone
Social anxiety	Decrease concentration and attention Cause significant distress or impairment in social, academic, occupational or any important area of functioning	The anxiety is about social situations and the focus is on fear of being negatively evaluated by others

Kooij et al. (2012) and APA (2013)

3.3.3 Describe Some of the Difficulties in Conducting Meta-Analysis on the Effect of Stimulant Medications on Comorbid Anxiety in ADHD Patients in the Current Literature?

Meta-analysis for the effect of stimulant medication on anxiety has been difficult to conduct for several reasons such as the use of different rating scales, different reporting methods, lack of numerical results obtained with rating scales or partial findings only.

3.3.4 List Some of the Instruments That Would Assist Clinicians in Identifying Different Anxiety Disorders?

Disorder	Scale	Reference
Generalized anxiety disorder	Multidimensional anxiety scale for children (MASC)	March et al. (1997)
Social anxiety	Liebowitz social anxiety scale foe children and adolescents	Tyrala et al. (2015)
	The *Social Phobia and Anxiety Scale for Children (SPAI-C)*	
	The *Social Anxiety Scale for Adolescents (SAS-A)*	La Greca and Lopez (1998)
Panic disorder	The panic disorder severity scale for children (PDSS-C)	Elkins et al. (2014)

Disorder	Scale	Reference
Phobia	Short form of the fear survey schedule for children-revised (FSSC-R-SF)	
Anxiety disorder	Screen for child anxiety related disorders (SCARED)	
	Multidimensional anxiety scale for children (MASC)	March et al. (1997)

3.3.5 What Is the Role of Parental Anxiety in Patients with ADHD and Anxiety?

Anxiety disorders more likely in parents and family (Pfiffner and McBurnett 2006; Kepley and Ostrander 2007).

More than 18% of parents have significant symptoms of anxiety or depression (Vidair et al. 2011).

Child and parental anxiety are associated with low rates of positive parental behavior, over-protectiveness of the child, less autonomy for the child, lower child self-sufficiency, and parent modeling of anxiety. The excessive parental control may increase child perceptions of threat, decrease children's sense of controlling threats, and decreased opportunity for experience with managing threats (Van der Bruggen et al. 2008).

3.3.6 Describe Some of the Literature Findings on the Relationship Between Trauma and ADHD?

Maltreatment has been considered common to children who have disabilities including ADHD diagnosis (Prayez et al. 2011). One study found that children with ADHD inattentive type are more likely to experience neglect, physical neglect, physical abuse and sexual abuse. ADHD hyperactive type was found to be related to neglect and physical abuse (Ouyang et al. 2008).

The rate of experience of any sexual abuse was 20.9% (28.7% for females and 13.3% for males) in a study that investigated 4910 students aged between 15 and 18 with ADHD (Sonnby et al. 2011).

History of any abuse was found to be higher in girls with ADHD than in controls (14.3 vs. 4.5%) (Briscoe-Smith and Hinshaw 2006).

From another aspect, ADHD, was the most common psychiatric comorbidity among the group of sexually, physically and emotionally abused children and the rate of comorbidity was 22% (Cengel-Kultur et al. 2007).

Overall, traumatic experiences during childhood are possibly associated with ADHD and anxiety disorders. Some authors suggest that relationship between trauma and anxiety and ADHD is complex and has not been studied extensively (Koyuncu et al. 2016).

3.3.7 What Are the Treatment Considerations in Comorbid ADHD and Anxiety Disorders?

Some authors raised concerns that stimulant medications may lead to exacerbation of anxiety disorders and sleep problems in patients with comorbid ADHD and anxiety disorders (Pliszka 1989; Van der Oord et al. 2008; Duong et al. 2012).

Some reports suggest that anxiety does not lessen response to ADHD stimulant treatment (Abikoff et al. 2005).

Combination of SSRI and stimulant medications have been combined successfully in the management of both conditions (Lavretsky et al. 2015; Koran et al. 2009).

Atomoxetine was found to be efficacious in reducing ADHD and anxiety symptoms in patients who had both conditions (Adler et al. 2009).

Non-pharmacological, psychosocial intervention may be a useful adjunct to pharmacotherapy in patients with ADHD and anxiety (Antshel et al. 2014; Houghton et al. 2017).

Anxiety disorders can present with symptoms consistent with ADHD. If there is no pre-morbid history of ADHD prior to onset of anxiety disorder may be a primary anxiety disorder and not co-morbid ADHD. Treatment should focus on anxiety disorder, and then once adequately treated can reassess for ADHD.

Multiple studies demonstrate the efficacy of a cognitive-behavioral therapy intervention (CBT) in the treatment of anxiety disorders and OCD in children and adolescents. CBT outcomes are not as good if parental anxiety remains high and/or if paternal rejection and depression are present. Family therapy may be helpful to increase family awareness of how anxiety is influenced within the family dynamics and to improve communication and anxiety/distress tolerance within the family. Parent Behavioral therapy (BT) focused on increasing positive parenting behavior support and reducing over-protectiveness and harsh discipline also has evidence of helping in ADHD (Liber et al. 2008).

Some guidelines recommend treating the most disabling disorder first. If clinicians start with ADHD treatment with a stimulant medication and the anxiety symptoms increase, then stimulant medication should be decreased or discontinued. Combination of SSRIs and stimulant medications are possible but frequent monitoring is required (CADDRA 2017).

Results of a Meta-analysis for comparative effectiveness and safety of cognitive behavioral therapy and pharmacotherapy for childhood anxiety disorders were recently published. It concludes that there is evidence supporting the effectiveness of CBT and SSRIs for reducing childhood anxiety symptoms. Serotonin-norepinephrine reuptake inhibitors also appear to be effective based on less consistent evidence. The review suggests there is a need for head-to-head comparisons between various medications and comparisons with CBT (Wang et al. 2017).

3.3.8 What Are the Dosing Recommendations for Atomexetine (ATX) in Children and Adolescents?

ATX can start at 10–20 mg and titrated to optimal dose (80 mg) over 11 weeks. The maximum daily dose approved by the US FDA for children and adolescents who weigh less than70 kg is 1.4 mg/kg/day; for children and adolescents who weigh 70 kg and adults, it is 100 mg/day.

Studies using up to 2.4 mg/kg/day and 3.0 mg/kg/day have not shown an improved overall response in children or adolescents who did not respond to lower doses of ATX (1.2–1.8 mg/kg/day) (Kratochvil et al. 2007).

3.3.9 What Are the Specific Tapering Recommendations to Stop Atomoxetine and What Are the Withdrawal Symptoms?

When discontinuing ATX, tapering is not necessary as stopping the medication is not associated with acute discontinuation symptoms (Wernicke et al. 2004).

3.3.10 What Are the Dosing Reduction Requirements in Adolescents with Hepatic Impairment When Prescribing Atomoxetine?

For subjects with hepatic impairment, the dose should be reduced to 50% of the normal dose for those with moderate impairment, and to 25% of the original dose for those with severe impairment (Kratochvil et al. 2007).

3.3.11 Does the Literature Recommends Fast Dose Titration or Slow Dose Titration When Starting Atomoxetine?

There is limited data. One study evaluated the effects of a daily dosing regimen and speed of titration in a post hoc analysis of 22 child/adolescent and found the following:

The time to the start of treatment-emergent adverse effects was significantly shorter in subjects who received once-a-day versus twice-a-day dosing. Time to onset of decreased appetite, abdominal pain, and somnolence significantly decreased with fast titration in children and adults.

Fast titration was defined as ATX 0.5 mg/kg/day × 7 days, then ATX 1.2 mg/kg/day versus slow titration ATX 0.5 mg/kg/day × 7 days, then ATX 0.8 mg/kg/day for 7 days, followed by ATX 1.2 mg/kg/day for children (Kratochvil et al. 2007).

References

Abikoff H, McGough J, Vitiello B, et al. RUPP ADHD/Anxiety Study Group. Sequential pharmacotherapy for children with comorbid attention-deficit/hyperactivity and anxiety disorders. J Am Acad Child Adolesc Psychiatry. 2005;44(5):418–27.

Adler LA, Liebowitz M, Kronenberger W, et al. Atomoxetine treatment in adults with attention-deficit/hyperactivity disorder and comorbid social anxiety disorder. Depress Anxiety. 2009;26(3):212–21.

American Psychiatric Association. Diagnostic and statistical manual of mental disorders. 5th ed. Washington, DC: American Psychiatric Association; 2013.

Antshel KM, Faraone SV, Gordon M. Cognitive behavioral treatment outcomes in adolescent ADHD. J Atten Disord. 2014;18(6):483–95.

Briscoe-Smith AM, Hinshaw SP. Linkages between child abuse and attention-deficit/hyperactivity disorder in girls: behavioral and social correlates. Child Abuse Negl. 2006;30:1239–55.

Canadian Attention Deficit Hyperactivity Disorder Resource Alliance (CADDRA). Canadian ADHD practice guidelines. 4th ed. Toronto, ON: CADDRA; 2017. WWW.CADDRA.CA.

Cengel-Kultur E, Cuhadaroglu-Cetin F, Gokler B. Demographic and clinical features of child abuse and neglect cases. Turk J Pediatr. 2007;49(3):256.

Duong S, Chung K, Wigal SB. Metabolic, toxicological, and safety considerations for drugs used to treat ADHD. Expert Opin Drug Metab Toxicol. 2012;8(5):543–52.

Elkins RM, Pincus DB, Comer JS. A psychometric evaluation of the panic disorder severity scale for children and adolescents. Psychol Assess. 2014;26(2):609–18.

Gadow K, et al. Comparative study of children with ADHD only, autism spectrum disorder + ADHD, and chronic multiple tic disorder + ADHD. J Atten Disord. 2009;12(5):474–85.

Houghton S, Alsalmi N, Tan C, Taylor M, Durkin K. Treating comorbid anxiety in adolescents with ADHD using a cognitive behavior therapy program approach. J Atten Disord. 2017;21(13):1094–104.

Kepley H, Ostrander R. Family characteristics of anxious ADHD children: preliminary results. J Atten Disord. 2007;10:317–23.

Kessler RC, Adler L, Barkley R, et al. The prevalence and correlates of adult ADHD in the United States: results from the National Comorbidity Survey Replication. Am J Psychiatry. 2006;163(4):716–23.

Kooij JJ, Huss M, Asherson P, et al. Distinguishing comorbidity and successful management of adult ADHD. J Atten Disord. 2012;16(5 suppl):3S–19S.

Koran LM, Aboujaoude E, Gamel NN. Double-blind study of dextroamphetamine versus caffeine augmentation for treatment-resistant obsessive-compulsive disorder. J Clin Psychiatry. 2009;70(11):1530–5.

Koyuncu A, Çelebi F, Ertekin E, Kök BE, Tükel R. Attention deficit and hyperactivity in social anxiety disorder: relationship with trauma history and impulsivity. Atten Defic Hyperact Disord. 2016;8(2):95–100.

Kratochvil CJ, Michelson D, Newcorn JH, et al. High-dose atomoxetine treatment of ADHD in youths with limited response to standard doses. J Am Acad Child Adolesc Psychiatry. 2007;46(9):1128–37.

La Greca AM, Lopez N. Social anxiety among adolescents: linkages with peer relations and friendships. J Abnorm Child Psychol. 1998;26:83–94.

Lavretsky H, Reinlieb M, St Cyr N, Siddarth P, Ercoli LM, Senturk D. Citalopram, methylphenidate, or their combination in geriatric depression: a randomized, double-blind, placebo-controlled trial. Am J Psychiatry. 2015;172(6):561–9.

Liber J, et al. Parenting and parental anxiety and depression as predictors of treatment outcome for childhood anxiety disorders: has the role of fathers been underestimated? J Clin Child Adolesc Psychol. 2008;37(4):747–58.

March JS, Parker JD, Sullivan K, Stallings P, Conners CK. The multidimensional anxiety scale for children (MASC): factor structure, reliability, and validity. J Am Acad Child Adolesc Psychiatry. 1997;36(4):554–65.

Ouyang L, Fang X, Mercy J, Perou R, Grosse SD. Attention-deficit/hyperactivity disorder symptoms and child maltreatment: a population-based study. J Pediatr. 2008;153(6):851–6.
Pfiffner L, McBurnett K. Family correlates of comorbid anxiety disorders in children with attention deficit/hyperactivity disorder. J Abnorm Child Psychol. 2006;34:725–35.
Pliszka SR. Effect of anxiety on cognition, behavior, and stimulant response in ADHD. J Am Acad Child Adolesc Psychiatry. 1989;28:882–7.
Prayez F, Wodon I, Van Hyfte S, Linkowski P. Attention-deficit/hyperactivity disorder (ADHD) and child maltreatment: a review. Rev Med Brux. 2011;33(2):75–86.
Reinke W, Ostrander R. Heterotyic and homotypic continuity: the moderating effects of age and gender. J Abnorm Child Psychol. 2008;36(7):1109–22.
Sonnby K, Åslund C, Leppert J, Nilsson KW. Symptoms of ADHD and depression in a large adolescent population: co-occurring symptoms and associations to experiences of sexual abuse. Nord J Psychiatry. 2011;65(5):315–22.
Tai YM, Gau CS, Gau SS, Chiu HW. Prediction of ADHD to anxiety disorders: an 11-year national insurance data analysis in Taiwan. J Atten Disord. 2013;17(8):660–9.
The MTA Cooperative Group. Multimodal treatment of children with ADHD. A 14-month randomized clinical trial of treatment strategies for attention-deficit/hyperactivity disorder. Arch Gen Psychiatry. 1999;56:1073–86.
Tyrala K, Seweryn M, Bonk M, Bulska W, Orszulak K, Bratek A, Krysta K. Evaluation of the utility of Liebowitz social anxiety scale and Barratt impulsiveness scale in the diagnosis of social anxiety, impulsivity and depression. Psychiatr Danub. 2015;27(Suppl 1):S223–6.
Van der Bruggen CO, et al. Research review: the relation between child and parent anxiety and parental control: a meta-analytic review. J Child Psychol Psychiatry. 2008;49(12):1257–69.
van der Oord S, Prins PJ, Oosterlaan J, et al. Treatment of attention deficit hyperactivity disorder in children: predictors of treatment outcome. Eur Child Adolesc Psychiatry. 2008;17:73–81.
Vidair HB, et al. Screening parents during child evaluations: exploring parent and child psychopathology in the same clinic. J Am Acad Child Adolesc Psychiatry. 2011;50(5):441–50.
Wang Z, Whiteside SPH, et al. Comparative effectiveness and safety of cognitive behavioral therapy and pharmacotherapy for childhood anxiety disorders: a systematic review and meta-analysis. JAMA Pediatr. 2017;171(11):1049–56.
Wernicke JF, Adler L, Spencer T, et al. Changes in symptoms and adverse events after discontinuation of atomoxetine in children and adults with attention deficit/hyperactivity disorder: a prospective, placebo-controlled assessment. J Clin Psychopharmacol. 2004;24(1):30–5.

ADHD and Obesity

4

4.1 Objectives

- Describe the relationship between ADHD and obesity and the possible hypothesis explaining that relationship.
- Describe the principals of management of adolescent patients with ADHD and obesity
- Describe some of the research findings of the mental health related problems associated with obesity in children and adolescents

4.2 ADHD and Obesity Literature Review Questions

4.2.1 Describe the Possible Relationship Between ADHD and Obesity?

Recent meta-analysis found statistically significant association between ADHD and obesity/overweight regardless of possible confounders. The pooled prevalence of obesity was increased by about 40% in children with ADHD compared with subjects without ADHD.

The review also showed that gender did not significantly affect the association between ADHD and obesity (Cortese et al. 2016).

Researchers support the link between ADHD symptoms and obesity. A model incorporating genetic, behavioral, and psychological factor was suggested to fit this association and concludes that individuals who have more ADHD symptoms and carry a genetic profile associated with greater DA activation in the brain reward areas appear more likely to overeat and, as a result, may be at increased risk of obesity.

That recent research supports the "reward surfeit" view of obesity and challenges the hypothesis that diminished DA levels account for ADHD symptom–adiposity association (Patte et al. 2016).

J. Sadek, *Clinician's Guide to ADHD Comorbidities in Children and Adolescents*,
https://doi.org/10.1007/978-3-319-45635-5_4

4.2.2 What Are Some of the Different Hypothesis That May Explain the Association Between ADHD and Obesity?

Researchers suggested that several possibilities arise (Cortese et al. 2016). The first hypothesis is that ADHD could increase the risk of obesity particularly with the impulsive and inattentive components of ADHD. Expression of impulsivity with poor inhibitory control could reinforce abnormal eating behaviors that, in turn, would increase the likelihood of obesity. Inattention and poor planning might cause difficulties in adhering to regular eating patterns and dietary regimens. It may also be associated with lack of awareness of food intake.

The hyperactive component of ADHD might not decrease the risk of obesity since it might not be a constant but rather modulated by the context. For example, energy expenditure decreases while watching television, and children with ADHD have been shown to watch more television and engage in less physical activity than comparison subjects without ADHD. In addition, hyperactivity linked to restless behaviors may also include abnormal eating patterns. The true effect of ADHD subtypes, ADHD symptom severity or frequency, and other variables (e.g., watching television, sedentary activity) related to ADHD and obesity cannot be confirmed because of the paucity of data.

The second hypothesis is that ADHD and obesity share common biological risk factors, including genetic variants. ADHD and obesity may share dopaminergic dysfunctions underpinning reward deficiency processing, but this understanding needs to be better evaluated. Interestingly, a "reward deficiency syndrome," characterized by insufficient dopamine-related natural reinforcement that leads to "unnatural" immediate rewards (such as inappropriate eating), has been reported in both ADHD and obesity. In addition, oxidative stress, which is linked to obesity, has also been associated with ADHD.

The third hypothesis is that obesity or factors associated with it cause or mimic ADHD. For example sleep-disordered breathing and shorter or later sleep have been reported to manifest with ADHD-like symptoms.

4.2.3 What Is the Impact of ADHD on Weight Loss Effort?

Compared to patients without ADHD, patients with ADHD had five times the number of previous weight loss attempts, more emotional eating, double the fast food consumption, and 31% who were able to lose 5% of their body weight compared to 61% in patients without ADHD (CADDRA 2015).

4.2.4 What Are the Principals of Management of Adolescent Patients with ADHD and Obesity?

Complete assessment of all ADHD comorbid disorders such as depression, anxiety, sleep disorders, obesity, and risk factors to determine the best order of treatment.

Multimodal treatment of ADHD should include psychosocial treatment and pharmacotherapy. Psychosocial treatment should also include psychoeducation on the interrelatedness of poor eating habits, late and short sleep, skipping meals, binge eating, and obesity. The ADHD symptoms of forgetfulness, poor planning, and impulsivity add to the complexity and longer duration of these behaviors. A patient's understanding of the relationship between factors may facilitate compliance for each step of treatment.

Treatment of comorbidity consists of treatment of the most severe disorder first, usually the mood disorder, with psychotherapy or pharmacotherapy as required. Melatonin may be added for the delayed sleep phase disorder to help reset the biological clock and lead to an earlier sleep onset and thus longer sleep duration. Sufficient sleep may improve mood and reduce carbohydrate craving, as well as the severity of ADHD symptoms.

Stimulant medications are usually recommended as the first line of line treatment (Pagoto et al. 2010). Pharmacological treatment for ADHD cannot be proven to decrease the risk of obesity associated with ADHD based on correlational studies. Overall, there is limited empirical evidence on the short- and long-term effects of psychostimulants on weight (Cortese et al. 2016). The improved planning of meals and the ability to keep to a diet seem to be the most important contributions of the stimulant treatment for weight loss. Weight loss as a side effect of stimulants is usually limited and not long lasting (Kooij 2016). ADHD treatment could also facilitate weight loss by improved self-directedness, improving day time energy, decreasing novelty seeking, and ability to pay attention to signals of hunger and satiety (Levy et al. 2009).

4.2.5 Describe Some of the Research Findings of the Mental Health Related Problems Associated with Obesity in Children and Adolescents?

One study suggests that children with obesity were less likely to complete ≥12 years in school (Hagman et al. 2017). Other Recent review (Rankin et al. 2016) suggested that overweight and obese children compared to normal-weight children had:

- Lower self-esteem, mood problems
- Poorer health related quality of life
- Multiple and clinically significant associated psychosocial problems such as disobedience, disruptive aggressive and destructive behavior, physical and verbal abuse, intense bullying and teasing, stigma and eating disorders.

References

CADDRA. 2015. WWW.CADDRA.CA.

Cortese S, Moreira-Maia CR, St Fleur D, Morcillo-Peñalver C, Rohde LA, Faraone SV. Association between ADHD and obesity: a systematic review and meta-analysis. Am J Psychiatry. 2016;173(1):34–43.

Hagman E, Danielsson P, Brandt L, Svensson V, Ekbom A, Marcus C. Childhood obesity, obesity treatment outcome, and achieved education: a prospective cohort study. J Adolesc Health. 2017;61(4):508–13.

Kooij JJ. ADHD and obesity. Am J Psychiatry. 2016;173(1):1–2.

Levy LD, Fleming JP, Klar D. Treatment of refractory obesity in severely obese adults following management of newly diagnosed attention deficit hyperactivity disorder. Int J Obes. 2009;33(3):326–34.

Pagoto SL, Curtin C, Bandini LG, Anderson SE, Schneider KL, Bodenlos JS, Ma Y. Weight loss following a clinic-based weight loss program among adults with attention deficit/hyperactivity disorder symptoms. Eat Weight Disord. 2010;15(3):e166–72.

Patte KA, Davis CA, Levitan RD, Kaplan AS, Carter-Major J, Kennedy JL. A behavioral genetic model of the mechanisms underlying the link between obesity and symptoms of ADHD. J Atten Disord. 2016. pii: 1087054715618793.

Rankin J, Matthews L, Cobley S, Han A, Sanders R, Wiltshire HD, Baker JS. Psychological consequences of childhood obesity: psychiatric comorbidity and prevention. Adolesc Health Med Ther. 2016;7:125–46.

ADHD and Oppositional Defiant Disorder (ODD) 5

5.1 Objectives

- Describe the diagnostic and management considerations of comorbid ADHD and ODD
- List some of the etiological risk factors associated with ODD
- List some of the instruments that would assist clinicians in identifying ADHD and ODD.
- Describe the prevalence rates and some epidemiological data of ADHD and ODD

5.2 The Case

Read the following case and check if the clinician completed the following tasks in this case?

- Obtained full psychiatric and medical history?
- Used some rating scales or questionnaires during the assessment?
- Obtained collateral history?
- Reviewed functional impairment?
- Conducted appropriate investigations, blood work and physical exam as indicated?
- Documented the assessment?
- Reached a diagnosis and assessed for comorbid disorders?
- Communicated results of the assessment to the patient and family?
- Provided adequate education to patient and family?
- Explained the possible pharmacological and psychosocial treatments and alternatives?
- Provided appropriate management and treatment interventions
- Explained the risk and benefit of treatment and lack of treatment?

J. Sadek, *Clinician's Guide to ADHD Comorbidities in Children and Adolescents*,
https://doi.org/10.1007/978-3-319-45635-5_5

- Referred the patient to other services or resources in the community as indicated?
- Suggested appropriate accommodations?
- Provided a follow up appointment?

5.2.1 Owen Oland

8 year old boy referred at request of the school because of very disruptive behavior. He had several detentions and was suspended twice from school.

5.2.2 History of Present Illness

Recent school reports were suggestive that Owen has been very defiant and refused to do his work in school. Parents are also concerned that he is disrespectful at home and aggressive with his younger brother. He enjoys playing with other children but often gets into fights and arguments. He blames his friends and parents but he never accepts responsibility for his actions. At home, he gets aggressive with his brother when his brother gets attention from the parents. He kicks and screams when his parents asks him to go to bed. If they insist that he needs to go to bed, he throws his toys to show his frustration.

Owen needs prompting in the morning to brush his teeth and get ready for school. He is easily distracted by the morning news and parents have to turn off the TV to get him to finish getting ready. Owen forgets to put his homework in his back pack and parents need to check that frequently.

Owen starts to argue if he cannot select his lunch sandwich and forces his mother to make him what he wants.

After school, he refuses to do his homework and his dad has to sit down with him to finish his homework after school. He loves Hockey but when he loses, he kicks his brother and blames his coach.

Owen has been constantly losing things in school such as his books. He interrupts others and talk over them. His parents also mentioned that he gets bored easily and has difficulty staying focused for more than few minutes.

Teachers had serious concerns particularly around disrupting the classroom and refusing to do tasks.

Owen never had any therapy and does not take any medications.

Screening for anxiety disorders, developmental or intellectual disability, specific learning disorder, mood disorder was unrevealing.

5.2.2.1 Medical History

Owen has no known drug allergies. He had no serious medical problems, surgery or hospitalizations.

No history of any major childhood illnesses and he received all her vaccinations appropriately in a timely fashion. Blood work did not reveal any abnormal findings. He has no active medical symptoms.

5.2.2.2 Family History

Owen's mother has been diagnosed with depression and has been stable on Citalopram 40 mg daily for 4 years. Father smokes weed regularly.

5.2.2.3 Personal and Developmental History

OO was the product of an uncomplicated pregnancy. He was born in Halifax, Nova Scotia. Delivery was on time and was a vaginal delivery.

Her developmental motor and language milestones were met in a timely manner.

He was born in intact family and has one younger brother (6). No history of physical, sexual, or emotional abuse or domestic violence.

Owen is popular and has lots of friends. He enjoys playing videogames.

5.2.2.4 Behavior in the Office

Owen was active in the office but was able to settle and answer questions. He said that he gets angry but blamed others for making him angry. He mentioned that all the problems are not his fault.

5.2.2.5 Case Outcome

Based on clinical assessment and information from both parents and the school, Owen was diagnosed with ADHD combined type and ODD. He responded well to behavioral therapy (BT), parenting coaching and Methylphenidate long acting 20 mg daily in the morning.

His blood pressure remained stable at 90/60 and pulse is 69. Height and weight were also monitored and remained within the growth curve.

5.3 Literature Review Questions

5.3.1 How Was the Diagnosis of ODD Made in This Case?

ODD is characterized by a pattern of negativistic, hostile and defiant behavior and can occur in one setting only, in which case it is deemed "mild"—this is most typically at home but can be at school. Thus, the behaviours do not need to be in more than one setting, unlike ADHD. In 2 settings, it is considered moderate and in 3 more settings, would be considered severe.

Symptoms should be lasting more than 6 months (before age 18), during which ≥4 (DSM-V) of the following are present for a significant period of time and cause significant impairment in functioning: angry and resentful, often loses temper, touchy/easily annoyed by others, argues with adults, often deliberately annoys people, actively defies/refuses to comply with adults' requests /rules, blames others for his/her mistakes/misbehaviors, spiteful/vindictive. The behaviors do not occur exclusively during the course of a psychotic, mood or substance use disorder. The behaviours also need to be exhibited with at least one individual who is not a sibling. Owen has more than 4 of the above symptoms that are displayed at home and at school.

5.3.2 Comment on the Epidemiology of ODD and the Comorbidity with ADHD?

The community prevalence of ODD is reported as ranging widely, between 1 and 16%, depending on which criteria and assessment methods are used, which time window is considered, and how many informants are used (Loeber et al. 2000).

Comorbidity rates of ADHD and ODD has been estimated around 40% based on the findings from the MTA cooperative study (MTA 1999).

Some data suggested that ODD occurs in up to 60% of individuals with ADHD (Connor and Doerfler 2008).

5.3.3 What Is the Natural Course of ODD?

The diagnosis of ODD is relatively stable over time, but most children (approximately 67%) will ultimately exit from the diagnosis after a 3-year follow-up (Connor 2002).

One third of children with early onset ODD progress to have conduct disorder (CD). 40% of kids with CD progress to have antisocial personality disorder in adulthood.

Although there is overlap between ODD and CD, CD involves the violation of others' basic rights or of age-appropriate norms and rules. ODD involves emotional symptoms, in addition to behavioural symptoms – these poorly controlled emotions, i.e. outbursts of anger, then go on to cause interpersonal difficulty. Only a minority of individuals with ODD develop CD (42.3%)" (Fonagy 2010).

5.3.4 Give Examples of Tools That Can be Used to Identify ADHD, Oppositional Defiant Disorder, and Other Behavioral Disorders?

SNAP 30 (Swanson, Nolan and Pelham Teacher and Parent Rating Scale)

The Strength and difficulties questionnaire

Connors rating scale (Connors Parent Rating Scale and Connors Teacher Rating Scale) (Conners et al. 1998)

Vanderbilt ADHD Diagnostic Parent Rating Scale

Child Behaviour Checklist (CBCL) with a construct for Internalizing and externalizing behaviors. It is 118 items used for School age and up and has good psychometrics and relies on Parent report (Achenbach 1991).

5.3.5 Mention Some of the Risk Factors Associated with ODD and ADHD?

Several risk factors have been identified as vulnerabilities that contribute to the development of ODD (Burke et al. 2002):

In utero exposure to toxins/drugs/alcohol, Low IQ, neuropsychological deficits, Difficult temperament, Lead poisoning, Learning disorder, Poor parent-child fit, Low socioeconomic status, abuse/maltreatment, and parental psychopathology.

Biological factors have small contribution in ODD, as there is familial clustering of ODD (Burke et al. 2002).

Temperamental factors have been implicated in the future development of disruptive behavior (Connor 2002; Burke et al. 2002).

Some variance in ODD severity is also related to disrupted parenting:

Inconsistent, indiscriminate, emotional, and episodically vacillating between harsh and permissive (lax) consequences teaches social coercion as a means of social interaction.

But timid parenting is the most important factor contributing to ODD which feeds back to make parents more reluctant to discipline.

Ineffective parenting can partly arise from parental ADHD and other high risk parental disorders in ADHD families (e.g., depression, ASP, SUDS).

Early ODD predicts persistence of ADHD and increases risk for enuresis, CD/MDD and anxiety.

Emotional dysregulation component predicts later MDD; conflict component predicts later CD.

Some researchers suggested an etiological model where the inherited characteristics of the child interact with the environment to produce symptoms and the parenting component of this environment may itself have genetic determinants.

Specific risk factors for ODD, compared with ADHD, include deviant peer affiliation, harsh or inconsistent parenting, low levels of parental affection, and exposure to family violence (Boden et al. 2010).

Recent European study that assessed three models investigating risk factors for ADHD-only versus controls, ADHD + ODD versus controls, and ADHD + ODD versus ADHD-only concluded that adverse life events and parental ADHD were risk factors for both ADHD + ODD and ADHD-only, and more adverse life events were an even stronger risk factor for comorbid ODD compared with ADHD-only.

For ADHD + ODD, but not ADHD-only, parental criticism, deviant peer affiliation, and parental SES acted as risk factors.

Maternal smoking during pregnancy acted as minor risk factor for ADHD-only, while higher birth weight acted as minor risk factor for ADHD + ODD (Noordermeer et al. 2017).

5.3.6 What Are the General Treatment Recommendations for ODD?

1. Establish therapeutic alliance with the child and family
2. Consider culture issues when diagnosing and treating ODD
3. Obtain information directly from the child and parents regarding symptoms, onset, duration and impairment
4. Consider carefully the psychiatric comorbidity when diagnosing and treating ODD
5. Include information from multiple outside informants if possible
6. Use questionnaires and rating scales in assessment of ODD and tracking progress
7. Develop individualized treatment plan based on the specific clinical situation
8. Select an evidence based parent intervention
9. Use medications as adjuncts to non-pharmacological treatment for comorbid disorders and symptomatic treatment
10. Consider intensive and prolonged treatment for severe and persistent ODD (AACAP 2007).

5.3.7 What Are the Psychosocial Management Recommendations for ODD?

1. Parental management training. Collaborative problem solving, in which parents and children work together, is an effective technique for treating ODD (Greene et al. 2004).
2. In schools, teachers' training for behavioral interventions
3. Peer group support and peer-mediated intervention
4. Social awareness and supervision
5. Cognitive behavior therapy (CBT): perspective taking, problem-solving skills training, assertive training, anger management training. Group CBT for children has also been found to decrease aggressive behaviors (Goertz-Dorten et al. 2017). Some researchers suggested that parenting interventions are needed for effective CBT treatment (Forehand et al. 2016).
6. Functional family therapy or brief strategic family therapy (Ghosh et al. 2017).
7. Individualized treatment plans by mental health professionals for both the child and family are the most effective. Behavioral parenting interventions are first-line therapy in younger children. In adolescence, individual therapy takes a more prominent role, but outcomes are better when parents are involved. Early intervention may help prevent other disorders, such as conduct disorder, substance abuse, and delinquency (Riley et al. 2016).

5.3.8 What Are the Treatment Considerations in Comorbid ADHD and ODD?

The treatment of ADHD and comorbid ODD involves management of the core symptoms of ADHD plus, in many cases, augmentation with other treatment (psychological or pharmacological) to manage ODD.

Both stimulants and ATX reduce the symptoms when it is comorbid with ADHD; not when ODD is alone. There is no evidence that one stimulant preparation is more effective than another for ADHD and comorbid ODD.

Higher doses may be needed for ODD comorbid with ADHD. Comorbid cases also require adjunctive parent training in behavior management methods (AACAP 2007).

The response may be related to age since the success rate for children is 60–75% and 25–35% for adolescents age 13 and above.

Some authors suggest treating parent's ADHD first and to add problem-solving communication training of teen and parents after age 14 years.

Recent, a review of digitally assisted parent training programs (DPTs) targeting the treatment of children and adolescents with disruptive Behaviors showed efficacy across a range of therapy formats applied in real-world settings. DPTs demonstrated the potential for increased accessibility of evidence- based treatment for youth with disruptive behaviors (Baumel et al. 2017).

In severe and persistent cases when intensive and prolonged treatment is needed, clinicians should select the least restrictive treatment setting that guarantees safety and regular delivery of interventions.

Day treatment, residential, and hospitalization facilities may need to be considered if the family is unable or unwilling to collaborate with the treatment of a more severe case of ODD. Hospitalizations are needed for crisis management only. Community-based alternatives to residential placement include therapeutic foster care and respite care (Chamberlain 2003).

5.3.8.1 For ADHD with Behavioural Problems

Methylphenidate/stimulants have best evidence followed by atomoxetine, and guanfacine SR, clonidine (Ghosh et al. 2017).

5.3.8.2 For Treatment of Aggression

- Antipsychotic (risperidone followed by aripiprazole has the best evidence, followed by other atypical and typical antipsychotics)
- In cases of partial response, mood stabilizer can be added
- For no response, antipsychotic can be changed (Ghosh et al. 2017)

5.3.9 List Some of the Parent Training Programs That Are Supported by Randomized Controlled Trials?

Incredible Years for ages up to 8 years of age. It can be administered in groups for parents, teachers and children and the website is http//:www.incredibleyears.com (Webster-Stratton et al. 2004).

Triple P-Positive Parenting Program for ages up to 13 years of age. A program for parents and the website is http://www.triplep-parenting.ca (Sanders et al. 2000).

Parent-Child Interactional Therapy for children up to 8 years of age. A program for parents and children and mode of administration is Individual and family. The website is http//:www.pcit.org (Brinkmeyer and Eyberg 2003).

Helping the Noncompliant Child: Parenting and Family Skills Program for ages up to 8 years of age. A program for parents and children and mode of administration is Individual and family (McMahon and Forehand 2003; Hough and Daniel 2003).

COPE program for ages up to 14 years. It is administered in groups for parents (Cunningham 1998; Cunningham et al. 1995).

Defiant Children for ages up to 12 years. It can be administered for Individuals or family (Barkley 1997, The Guilford Press).

The Adolescent Transitions Program (ATP) for ages up to 13 years. A program for parents and children and administered as Individual, family or in groups. The website is https://www.childtrends.org/programs/adolescent-transitions-program-comprehensive/(Dishion et al. 2003; Dishion and Kavanagh 2002).

References

AACAP. Practice parameter for the assessment and treatment of children and adolescents with attention-deficit/hyperactivity disorder. J Am Acad Child Adolesc Psychiatry. 2007;46:894–921.

Achenbach TM. Manual for child behavior checklist 4Y18, 1991 profile. Burlington, VT: Department of Psychiatry; 1991.

Barkley RA. Defiant children, second edition: a Clinician's manual for assessment and parent training. New York: The Guilford Press; 1997.

Baumel A, Pawar A, Mathur N, Kane JM, Correll CU. Technology-assisted parent training programs for children and adolescents with disruptive behaviors: a systematic review. J Clin Psychiatry. 2017;78(8):e957–69.

Boden JM, Fergusson DM, Horwood LJ. Risk factors for conduct disorder and oppositional/defiant disorder: evidence from a New Zealand birth cohort. J Am Acad Child Adolesc Psychiatry. 2010;49:1125–33.

Brinkmeyer M, Eyberg SM. Parent-child interaction therapy for oppositional children. In: Kazdin AE, Weisz JR, editors. Evidence-based psychotherapies for children and adolescents. New York: The Guilford Press; 2003. p. 204–23.

Burke JD, Loeber R, Birmaher B. Oppositional defiant disorder and conduct disorder: a review of the past 10 years, part II. J Am Acad Child Adolesc Psychiatry. 2002;41:1275–93.

Chamberlain P. An overview of the history and development of the multidimensional treatment foster care model and the supporting research. In: Chamberlain P, editor. Treating chronic juvenile offenders: advances made through the Oregon multidimensional treatment Foster Care model. Law and public policy. Washington, DC: American Psychological Association; 2003. p. 47Y67.

Conners CK, Sitarenios G, Parker JD, Epstein JN. The revised Conners_parent rating scale (CPRS-R): factor structure, reliability, and criterion validity. J Abnorm Child Psychol. 1998;26:257Y268.

Connor DF. Aggression and antisocial behavior in children and adolescents: research and treatment. New York: The Guilford Press; 2002.

Connor DF, Doerfler LA. ADHD with comorbid oppositional defiant disorder or conduct disorder: discrete or nondistinct disruptive behavior disorders? J Atten Disord. 2008;12:126–34.

Cunningham CE. A large-group community-based, family systems approach to parent training. In: Barkley RA, editor. Attention-deficit/hyperactivity disorder: a handbook for diagnosis and treatment. New York: The Guilford Press; 1998. p. 394–412.

Cunningham CE, Bremner R, Boyle M. Large group community based parenting programs for families of preschoolers at risk for disruptive behaviour disorders: utilization, cost effectiveness, and outcome. J Child Psychol Psychiatry. 1995;36:1141–59.

Dishion TJ, Kavanagh K. The adolescent transitions program: a family-centered prevention strategy for schools. In: Reid JB, Snyder JJ, Patterson GR, editors. Antisocial behavior in children and adolescents: a developmental analysis and the Oregon model for intervention. Washington, DC: American Psychological Association; 2002. p. 257–72.

Dishion TJ, Nelson SE, Kavanagh K. The family check-up for high risk adolescents: motivating parenting monitoring and reducing problem behavior. Special series: behavior oriented interventions for children with aggressive behavior and/or conduct problems. Behav Ther. 2003;34:553Y571.

Fonagy P. Psychotherapy research: do we know what works for whom? Br J Psychiatry. 2010;197(2):83–5.

Forehand R, Parent J, Sonuga-Barke E, Peisch VD, Long N, Abikoff HB. Which type of parent training works best for preschoolers with comorbid ADHD and ODD? A secondary analysis of a randomized controlled trial comparing generic and specialized programs. J Abnorm Child Psychol. 2016;44(8):1503–13.

Ghosh A, Ray A, Basu A. Oppositional defiant disorder: current insight. Psychol Res Behav Manag. 2017;10:353–67.

Goertz-Dorten A, Benesch C, Hautmann C, et al. Efficacy of an individualized social competence training for children with oppositional defiant disorders/conduct disorders. Psychother Res. 2017;27(3):326–37.

Greene RW, Ablon JS, Goring JC, et al. Effectiveness of collaborative problem solving in affectively dysregulated children with oppositional-defiant disorder: initial findings. J Consult Clin Psychol. 2004;72(6):1157–64.

Hough MG, Daniel SS. Parenting the strong-willed child: the clinically proven five-week program for parents of two- to six-year-olds. J Am Acad Child Adolesc Psychiatry. 2003;42:1380–1.

Loeber R, Burke JD, Lahey BB, Winters A, Zera M. Oppositional defiant and conduct disorder: a review of the past 10 years, part I. J Am Acad Child Adolesc Psychiatry. 2000;39(12):1468–84.

McMahon RR, Forehand RL. Helping the noncompliant child. New York: The Guilford Press; 2003.

MTA Cooperative Group. Moderators and mediators of treatment response for children with attention-deficit/hyperactivity disorder. Arch Gen Psychiatry. 1999;56:1088Y1096.

Noordermeer SDS, Luman M, Weeda WD, Buitelaar JK, Richards JS, Hartman CA, Hoekstra PJ, Franke B, Heslenfeld DJ, Oosterlaan J. Risk factors for comorbid oppositional defiant disorder in attention-deficit/hyperactivity disorder. Eur Child Adolesc Psychiatry. 2017;26(10):1155–64.

Riley M, Ahmed S, Locke A. Common questions about oppositional defiant disorder. Am Fam Physician. 2016;93(7):586–91.

Sanders MR, Markie-Dadds C, Tully L, Bor B. The triple PY positive parenting program: a comparison of enhanced, standard, and self-directed behavioural family intervention for parents of children with early onset conduct problems. J Consult Clin Psychol. 2000;68:624–40.

Webster-Stratton C, Reid MJ, Hammond M. Treating children with early-onset conduct problems: intervention outcomes for parent, child, and teacher training. J Clin Child Adolesc Psychol. 2004;33:105–24.

6 ADHD and Conduct Disorder (CD)

6.1 Objectives

- Describe the prevalence rates and morbidity associated with Attention Deficit Hyperactivity Disorder (ADHD) and Conduct Disorder comorbidity
- List some of the etiological risk factors associated with Conduct Disorder
- Describe the diagnostic and management considerations of comorbid ADHD and Conduct Disorder

6.2 The Case

Read the following case and check if the clinician completed the following tasks in this case?

- Obtained full psychiatric and medical history?
- Used some rating scales or questionnaires during the assessment?
- Obtained collateral history?
- Reviewed functional impairment?
- Conducted appropriate investigations, blood work and physical exam as indicated?
- Documented the assessment?
- Reached a diagnosis and assessed for comorbid disorders?
- Communicated results of the assessment to the patient and family?
- Provided adequate education to patient and family?
- Explained the possible pharmacological and psychosocial treatments and alternatives?
- Provided appropriate management and treatment interventions
- Explained the risk and benefit of treatment and lack of treatment?

J. Sadek, *Clinician's Guide to ADHD Comorbidities in Children and Adolescents*,
https://doi.org/10.1007/978-3-319-45635-5_6

- Referred the patient to other services or resources in the community as indicated?
- Suggested appropriate accommodations?
- Provided a follow up appointment?

6.3 Alex Alexander

6.3.1 Identifying Information

Alex is a 17 year old boy who lives with his parents (Father 40 and Mother 38) and younger brother in Moncton, NB, Canada.

Three months ago, Alex was were accused of committing an armed robbery within a home in Moncton and had some jail time while awaiting court.

The court requested a mental health assessment.

6.3.2 Charges Related to the Incident

Robbery, Possess weapon dangerous to public, assault with a weapon, pointing a firearm, careless use of firearm or weapon.

6.3.3 History of Present Illness

The patient has a long history of mental illness. He was bullied daily in junior high school. He struggled academically and socially in school since grade primary. He has multiple difficulties related to inattention, hyperactivity and impulsivity.

He was actually diagnosed with ADHD in 2006 at age 5 by his pediatrician.

In terms of ADHD parents and patient confirmed a long history that started in childhood and persisted in multiple settings of the following symptoms:

Fails to give close attention to details or makes careless mistakes in tasks
Has difficulty sustaining attention in tasks (few minutes)
Does not seem to listen when spoken to directly (frequent day dreaming)
Does not follow through on instructions and fails to finish school work, chores, or duties (persistent and frequent. Needs daily frequent reminders)
He is extremely disorganized in his home and school life.
Avoids, dislikes, or reluctantly engages in tasks requiring sustained mental effort (homework was a frequent struggle)
Loses things necessary for activities (mom could name many things)
Easily distracted by extraneous stimuli such as noise or movement.
Forgetful in daily activities (needs reminders)

Fidgets with hands or feet or squirms in seat (evident in the interview)
Runs about in situations in which it is inappropriate (instead of walking)
Had difficulty engaging in leisure activities quietly (as a child can get very loud).
Does things impulsively and without thinking
Interrupt others and has difficulty waiting his turn.

6.3.3.1 Substance Use

He started using alcohol in grade 9 when he was 15, then Cocaine age 16. He used acid once 6 month ago. He has been using weed daily for the past few years (1–2 g daily).

6.3.3.2 Mood Symptoms

Patient reported the following symptoms for the past 6 month:

Little interest or pleasure in things that he enjoyed such as snowboarding. He said he has been feeling low, and depressed, He had trouble falling or staying asleep. His energy level has been low and reported feeling tired, fatigued.

He was overeating and both parents confirmed that. His concentration is poor and has been fidgety and restless.

Alex has considered killing himself on different occasions and he specifically told his mother he will kill himself when he came out of jail. During the psychiatric assessment, he contracted for safety and promised he will not act on these dark thoughts to kill himself. There was no evidence of manic symptoms.

6.3.3.3 Anxiety Symptoms

He is an anxious individual but his anxiety became much worse while in jail.

His worries are present most days and was evident as a child. His mother said that he is very nervous or unable to relax most of the time. He had unexplained aches, headaches for the past year. He avoids social situations and worries a lot about people criticizing him.

In terms of Oppositional Defiant Disorder (ODD) parents reported:

He is often angry and resentful, often argues with his parents, often deliberately does things that annoy his brother but he is not easily annoyed by others. He argues with his teachers and parents and refuses to comply with adult rules.

In terms of CD, parents confirmed the following symptoms:

He can bully, threaten, or intimidate others.

He allegedly used a gun to threaten a person to obtain drugs recently.

Has never been physically cruel to animals.

He had deliberately destroyed others' property.

He stole from people's cars. Has several charges including robbery, armed robbery, using firearms.

He was involved in selling weed for 1 month.

Initiated few physical fights since he was in grade 6.

Have been physically cruel to people and broken into someone else's house (age 9).

Court report has significant details about many of these offenses.

6.3.4 Medical History

No medication allergy.

Current weight 160 lbs, height 5′9″.

- Alex had a concussion after falling in the house and hitting his head as a child.
- He had difficulty sleeping for 4 years from age 6–10 and was prescribed medications.
- In 2006, He was seen by a pediatrician who diagnosed him with **ADHD combined type** and started him on Ritalin.
- Another paediatrician continued to follow him and sent him for cardiac investigations after an EKG showed right bundle block in 2010 but he was asymptomatic and was medically cleared later. She continued to see him and prescribed him Concerta (MPH) 36 mg daily. He was receiving resource in Math and Language Arts. He was also seen by a psychologist who noted the diagnosis of **severe learning disability.**
- In grade 6 he received direct speech and language therapy for both expressive and receptive language disorder. The speech therapist made recommendations for further intervention in Junior high school since he did not show much progress.
- His mother took him to a naturopath in 2014 as she is not supportive of medications.

6.3.4.1 Past Psychiatric History

- Patient was seen by a psychologist more than a month prior to the incident. He was struggling in school. He was also experiencing other mental health symptoms such as low mood.
- At age 10, he saw the house directly across the street from his home demolished by fire. He has had traumatic memories related to the incident since that time.
- In 2008, he had psychoeducational assessment that indicated that Alex he met criteria for severe learning disability.

6.3.4.2 Family History

- He has an older step sister. Mother was 17 when she became pregnant with her.
- Maternal grandfather is alcoholic,
- Mom was diagnosed with generalized anxiety disorder and had depression when she was in her teens but refused medications.
- Maternal grandfather had bipolar disorder.
- Father had depression and anxiety.
- Sister had depression.
- Maternal grandfather and maternal great grandfather both were physically abusive.

6.3.5 Personal and Developmental History

There were no complications with mother's pregnancy.

The delivery was a vaginal delivery in Berlin, Germany.

His birth weight was 8 pounds 3 ounces. There were no neonatal concerns and went home at 2 days of age. He was bottle fed and his immunizations were up-to-date.

Patient had neither gross nor fine motor problems/difficulties. According to his parents.

Patient was assessed by a speech language pathologist in grade 6.

People notice odd behaviour with the child at age 4.

He was being bullied in junior high and that bullying played a major role in his poor self-esteem and need to be powerful and liked as stated by his father.

He said that he felt neglected by his parents as a child and they gave more attention to his 12 year old brother and 20 year old sister.

6.3.5.1 Interpersonal Relationships

Alex is not close to his parents. He has few good friends. He has one friend that he kept for 4 years. He had a supportive girlfriend at age 15 but he left her after 3 month.

6.3.5.2 School Information

Currently patient should be in Grade 11. He completed grade 10.

Past school grades had been poor. Past school behaviour has been fair.

Alex had the following difficulties at school:

Suspension for hitting a teacher, incomplete homework, learning problems particularly reading and writing, detentions in junior high, poor grades, teased or picked on (This has been a very significant issue), speech problems.

He had attendance problems in high school, bad peer influence.

Had to repeat grade 11 but did half only. Patient has received Special Education services.

He had the following documented adaptation:

Environmental Strategies: Provided appropriate seating such as proximity, study carrel, etc.

Seated at the front to facilitate frequent check-ins and reduce distractions.

Student benefits from being near the front and away from distractions (windows, friends etc.).

Specific Adaptation(s): adapted to quizzes/tests/exams: Reduced multiple choice options, word banks without extra words, extra prompts/diagrams provided.

Provide multi step directions, Provide extra time to complete assessment, provided with organizational Strategies, Frequent check ins.

Adjust length/complexity/timeline of assignments.

Administer alternative assessment format(s), i.e., oral, audio CD, etc.

6.3.5.3 Mental Status Examination

Patient looks his stated age. He is appropriately dressed and groomed. Some psychomotor retardation. His affect is constricted, and his mood is low 2/10. No reactivity in his affect. His speech is low volume and monotonous. He has no formal thought disorder. He is thinking of killing himself but no plan and no intent. No evidence of delusions nor perceptual disturbances. He has no intent of acting on it. His insight is limited and his judgment is poor. He was alert, oriented × 3. He completed Connors continuous performance testing.

6.3.5.4 Impression

Alex is a 17 year old man with significant history of poor cognitive, academic and social functioning. He has multiple adversity factors that perpetuate his condition including non-compliance with medications. He also has a biological predisposition to mental illness due to his family history.

He met the following diagnostic criteria:

- History of specific learning disorder (reading, writing)
- History of Language disorder (expressive and receptive)
- Conduct disorder
- Oppositional Defiant Disorder
- ADHD combined type (F 90.2)
- Cannabis use disorder (F 12.20)

Plan: Alex was referred patient to a psychologist to help him with mood and anxiety symptoms. He was also restarted on stimulant medications. He was given a trial of Lysdexamfetamine (Vyvanse) 20 mg po AM daily and was provided with psychoeducation.

He was enrolled in a correction program and was also mandated to see an addiction counsellor while in jail.

6.4 Literature Review Questions

6.4.1 How Was the Diagnosis of Conduct Disorder Made in This Case?

According to the DSM-5, conduct disorder is defined as a repetitive and persistent pattern of behaviour that violates the basic rights of others or violates major age-appropriate societal rules or norms (American Psychiatric Association 2013). In the preceding 12 months, at least three out of 15 criteria must be present from any of the following four categories, with at least one criterion present in the last 6 months: aggression towards people or animals; destruction of property; deceitfulness or theft; or serious violation of rules.

The behavioural disturbances must also cause clinically significant impairment in social, academic or occupational functioning. Conduct disorder can be classed as mild, moderate or severe.

It is also categorized into childhood onset, adolescent onset and unspecified onset subgroups. The early onset group is believed to have a poorer prognosis with a more persistent course and more pervasive disturbances.

A specifier was added in DSM-5 for people with limited "prosocial emotion", showing callous and unemotional traits as research showed they tend to have a relatively more severe form of the disorder and a different treatment response (American Psychiatric Association 2013).

6.4.2 Describe Some of the Findings of Epidemiological Studies of Conduct Disorder?

Some researchers suggest that 5% of children and young people aged 5–15 years met the criteria for Conduct Disorder (Green et al. 2005; Kessler et al. 2012).

The gender ratio is approximately 2.5 males for each female. Males have more severe and frequent conduct problems (Pullatz and Bierman 2004).

Onset of Conduct Disorder prior to age 10 predicts continuation through childhood. Those with early onset have a lower IQ, more ADHD symptoms, lower neuropsychological tests Scores, greater peer difficulties and are more likely to come from dysfunctional family backgrounds (Moffitt 2006).

Early onset Conduct Disorder also predicts poorer adult outcomes in domains of violence, mental health, substance misuse, work and family life (Moffitt 2006).

6.4.3 What Are Some of the Risk Factors for Developing Conduct Disorder?

Risk factors include low school achievement, impulsiveness, parental contact with the criminal justice system, parental mental health or substance misuse problems, child abuse, low family income and little education (NICE 2013).

6.4.4 List Some of the Instruments Measuring Externalizing Mental Health Problems in Young People?

NIMH Diagnostic Interview Schedule for Children Version Four (NIMH DISC-IV): It is a structured diagnostic interview designed to address more than 30 psychiatric diagnoses that occur in children and adolescents. It has two parallel versions: the Youth version (DISC-C) has been designed for administration to children between the ages of 9 and 17 and

The Parent version (DISC-P) to parents or knowledgeable caretakers of children, aged 6 through 17 years.

Behavior Assessment System for Children, 2nd Edition BASC-2 (3rd addition is also available)

It is broad band behavior rating scale and has a comprehensive set of rating scales and forms including the Teacher Rating Scales (TRS), Parent Rating Scales (PRS), Self-Report of Personality (SRP), Student Observation System (SOS), and Structured Developmental History (SDH). Together, they help you understand the behaviors and emotions of children and adolescents. Teachers or other qualified observers can complete forms at three age levels—preschool (ages 2–5), child (ages 6–11), and adolescent (ages 12–21)—in about 10–20 min (Reynolds and Kamphaus 2004).

Child Behavior Checklist (CBCL). It is a standardized parent report on children's problem behavior. Considered broad band. The Child Behavior Checklist (CBCL; Achenbach and Rescorla 2001), now called the Achenbach System of Empirically Based Assessment, is a parent report form to screen for emotional, behavioral, and social problems. The CBCL's questions are associated with problems on a syndrome scale in eight different categories: anxious/depressed, withdrawn/depressed, somatic complaints, social problems, thought problems, attention problems, rule-breaking behavior, and aggressive behavior (Achenbach and Ruffle 2000).

Psychopathy Checklist-Youth Version (PCL-YV) (Jones et al. 2006). The Hare Psychopathy Checklist: Youth Version (PCL:YV) semi-structured interview and collateral information that can be used to help clinicians understand the factors that contribute to the development of adult antisocial behavior and psychopathy. Developed by Adelle E. Forth, PhD, David S. Kosson, PhD and Robert D. Hare, PhD.

Comprehensive Adolescent Severity Inventory (CASI). (Meyers et al. 2006) a self-report instrument assessing chemical dependency, psychosocial functioning, delinquency and risk behaviors (Meyers et al. 1995).

The Massachusetts Youth Screening instrument (MAYSI). It is a self-report instrument, specifically designed to assess mental health symptoms among youth in the juvenile justice system, and includes constructs such as alcohol and drug use and angry and irritable moods (Grisso et al. 2001).

The Strength and Difficulty Questionnaire- SDQ (Goodman 1997). Free at www.sdqinfo.org

It is a brief emotional and behavioural screening questionnaire for children and young people. The tool can capture the perspective of children and young people, their parents and teachers.

There are currently three versions of the SDQ: a short form, a longer form with an impact supplement (which assesses the impact of difficulties on the child's life) and a follow-up form. The 25 items in the SDQ comprise 5 scales of 5 items each. The scales include:

1. Emotional symptoms subscale
2. Conduct problems subscale
3. Hyperactivity/inattention subscale
4. Peer relationships problem subscale
5. Prosocial behaviour subscale

The Eyberg Child Behavior Inventory (ECBI) (Eyberg and Pincus 1999). The Eyberg Child Behavior Inventory (ECBI) is a parent rating scale that assesses child behavior problems using two scales: the intensity scale and the problem scale. The intensity scale is seen as the more objective scale, as it measures how frequent particular behaviors occur within the child, while the problem scale measures whether or not the parent sees that behavior as a problem.

The Sutter–Eyberg Student Behavior Inventory (SESBI-R) (Eyberg and Pincus 1999). The SESBI-R is a teacher-report measure used to assess conduct problems in youth ages 2–16. It contains 38 items that are rated on both Intensity and Problem scales. Teachers are able to indicate the current frequency of behavior problems and determine whether or not they find the behaviors to be problematic. The SESBI-R can be used in conjunction with the Eyberg Child Behavior Inventory (ECBI).

Other instruments exist such as the Overt Aggression Scale Modified (OAS-M) Scale, Aberrant Behaviour Checklist (ABC), The Revised Conflict Tactics Scale (Straus et al. 1996), Child Hostility Scale (Knight et al. 1994), Revised Behavior Problem Checklist (RBPC) (Curtis and Schmidt 1993).

6.4.5 What Are the Associated Features of Early Versus Late Onset Conduct Disorder?

Early onset Conduct Disorder may be associated with the following:

- Possible deficits in executive function
- Low intelligence
- Callous-unemotional traits,
- Impulsivity, and fearlessness and emotional over-reactivity
- Greater family dysfunction
- Low Socioeconomic status and poor house hold
- Aggression and 10 to 1 ratio of male to female
- Higher likelihood of progression to adult antisocial behavior and persistence of symptoms
- Symptoms developed due interaction between difficult temperament and dysfunctional or inadequate parenting leading to problems in emotional regulation, poor executive control of behavior, or problems in conscience development

In late onset:

- Males are 1.5 times more likely than females to exhibit late onset CD
- No clear neuropsychological deficits but character may have rebelliousness and rejecting of traditional status hierarchies.
- Higher likelihood of remission in adulthood
- Exaggeration/disruption of the developmental process of adolescent identity formation and delinquent peer affiliations (Frick and Viding 2009; Barry et al. 2013).

6.4.6 List Some Psychiatric Disorders That Can Be Included in the Differential Diagnosis of Conduct Disorder?

- ADHD
- Adjustment disorder with disturbance of conduct
- Mood Disorders: Depression or Bipolar Disorder. Anxiety disorders.
- Pervasive developmental disorders
- Antisocial personality disorder (above age 18) (NICE guidelines)

6.4.7 What Are Some of the Factors Predicting Poor Outcome in Conduct Disorder?

- ADHD
- Lower IQ
- Early onset of severe problems, before 8 years old
- Antisocial acts which are severe, frequent and varied
- Parental criminality; parental alcoholism
- Harsh, inconsistent parenting with high criticism, low warmth, low involvement and low supervision
- Poor socioeconomic status in poor neighborhood (NICE guideline 2013)

6.4.8 What Are the Comorbidity Rates of ADHD and Conduct Disorder (CD)?

ADHD and Conduct Disorders are highly comorbid, with a meta-analysis finding rates of CD in individuals with ADHD ranging from 3.1 to 41.0% and rates of ADHD in individuals with CD ranging from 13.9 to 100% (Angold et al. 1999).

6.4.9 What Are Some of the Research Findings on Long-Term Outcomes of ADHD and Conduct Disorder?

A meta-analysis of 98 studies looking at broad health and psychosocial outcomes associated with ADHD and Conduct Disorders experienced during childhood and adolescence suggested that the comorbidity is associated with disability beyond immediate health loss.

It includes poor academic achievement (e.g. failure to complete high school), other mental and substance use disorders (e.g. depression), criminality (e.g. arrest), employment related problems (e.g., unemployment).

The study demonstrated the importance of addressing ADHD and CD early in life to potentially decrease a wide range of future adverse outcomes (Erskine et al. 2016). The societal cost for youth with severe CD behaviors is estimated to be ten times higher than those without antisocial problems (Scott et al. 2001), and as a result it is important to diagnose and manage this condition (Erskine et al. 2016).

6.4.10 What Are the Selective Prevention Interventions for at Risk Children and Adolescents That May Reduce the Likelihood of Developing a Conduct Disorder?

Classroom-based emotional learning and problem-solving programs may be helpful and should be provided in a positive atmosphere and consist of interventions intended to:

- increase children's awareness of their own and others' emotions
- teach self-control of arousal and behavior
- promote a positive self-concept and good peer relations
- improve children's problem-solving skills.

Typically the programs should consist of up to 30 classroom-based sessions over the course of one school year (NICE 2013).

6.4.11 What Are the Psychosocial and Pharmacological Treatment Recommendations for Conduct Disorder and ADHD?

6.4.11.1 Psychosocial Interventions

Behavioural and cognitive-behavioural group-based parenting interventions (both parents) are effective and cost-effective for improving child conduct problems, parental mental health and parenting skills in the short term (Furlong et al. 2013).

Some guidelines for treatment of conduct disorder suggest parent or parent and child training programs done in group or individualized format. Group social and cognitive problem-solving programs can be offered to individuals above age 9.

Multimodal treatment should involve the child or young person and their parents and should have an explicit and supportive family focus and be based on a social learning model with interventions provided at individual, family, school, and criminal justice and community levels (NICE 2013).

6.4.11.2 Pharmacological Treatment

Stimulant medications or atomoxetine or Guanfacine XR, either as monotherapy or combined should be offered to patients with ADHD and CD. The level of aggression should be documented prior to starting treatment (Ghosh et al. 2017).

Recent meta-analysis suggested that the short term risperidone may reduce aggression and conduct problems in children and youths with disruptive behaviour disorders above age 5. Adverse effects should be monitored such as metabolic (including weight gain and diabetes), extrapyramidal (including akathisia, dyskinesia and dystonia), cardiovascular (including prolonging the QT interval), hormonal (including increasing plasma prolactin) and other adverse effects (Loy 2017). The clinician should review the effects of risperidone after 3–4 weeks and discontinue it if there is no indication of a clinically important response at 6 weeks (NICE 2013).

For the general treatment of aggression:

- An antipsychotic (generally after failure of psychosocial treatment): Risperidone followed by aripiprazole has the best evidence, followed by other atypical and typical antipsychotics.
- In cases of partial response, mood stabilizer can be added
- For no response, antipsychotic can be changed (Ghosh et al. 2017)
- Evidence supporting the use of divalproex in aggressive youth with ODD or CD is of low quality. Carbamazepine was no different from placebo for the management of aggression in youth with

For Treatment of comorbid anxiety/mood issues, addition of an antidepressant such as an SSRI or psychotherapy would be helpful.

References

Achenbach TM, Ruffle TM. The child behavior checklist and related forms for assessing behavioral/emotional problems and competencies. Pediatr Rev. 2000;21:265–71.

Achenbach TM, Rescorla LA. Manual for the ASEBA Preschool Forms and Profiles. Burlington, VT: University of Vermont, Research Center for Children, Youth, & Families; 2001.

American Psychiatric Association. Diagnostic and statistical manual of mental disorders (DSM-5). 5th ed. Arlington, VA: American Psychiatric Publishing; 2013.

Angold A, Costello EJ, Erkanli A. Comorbidity. J Child Psychol Psychiatry. 1999;40:57–87.

Barry CT, et al. Evidence-based assessment of conduct disorder: current considerations and preparation for DSM-5. Professional Psychol Res Pract. 2013;44:56.

Curtis PA, Schmidt LL. A Spanish translation of the revised behavior problem checklist. Child Welfare. 1993;72:453–60.

Erskine HE, Norman RE, Ferrari AJ, Chan GC, Copeland WE, Whiteford HA, Scott JG. Long-term outcomes of attention-deficit/hyperactivity disorder and conduct disorder: a systematic review and meta-analysis. J Am Acad Child Adolesc Psychiatry. 2016;55(10):841–50.

Eyberg SM, Pincus D. Eyberg child behavior inventory and sutter-eyberg student behavior inventory: professional manual. Odessa, FL: Psychological Assessment Resources; 1999.

Frick PJ, Viding E. Antisocial behavior from a developmental psychopathology perspective. Dev Psychopathol. 2009;21:1111–31.

Furlong M, McGilloway S, Bywater T, Hutchings J, Smith SM, Donnelly M. Cochrane review: behavioural and cognitive-behavioural group-based parenting programmes for early-onset conduct problems in children aged 3 to 12 years (review). Evid Based Child Health. 2013;8(2):318–692.

Ghosh A, Ray A, Basu A. Oppositional defiant disorder: current insight. Psychol Res Behav Manag. 2017;10:353–67.

Goodman R. The Strengths and Difficulties Questionnaire: a research note. J Child Psychol Psychiatry. 1997;38:581–6.

Green H, McGinnity A, Meltzer H, Ford T, Goodman R. Mental health of children and young people in Great Britain, 2004: summary report. Newport: Office for National Statistics; 2005.

Grisso T, Barnum R, Fletcher KE, Cauffman E, Peuschold D. Massachusetts youth screening instrument for mental health needs of juvenile justice youths. J Am Acad Child Adolesc Psychiatry. 2001;40:541–8.

Jones S, Cauffman E, Miller JD, Mulvey E. Investigating different factor structures of the psychopathy checklist: youth version: confirmatory factor analytic findings. Psychol Assess. 2006;18:33–48.

Kessler RC, Avenevoli S, Costello E, et al. Prevalence, persistence, and Sociodemographic correlates of DSM-IV disorders in the National Comorbidity Survey Replication Adolescent Supplement. Arch Gen Psychiatry. 2012;69(4):372–80.

Knight GP, Virdin LM, Ocampo KA, Roosa M. An examination of the cross-ethnic equivalence of measures of negative life events and mental health among hispanic and Anglo-American children. Am J Community Psychol. 1994;22:767–83.

Loy JH, Merry SN, Hetrick SE, Stasiak K. Atypical antipsychotics for disruptive behaviour disorders in children and youths. Cochrane Database Syst Rev. 2017;8:CD008559. https://doi.org/10.1002/14651858.

Meyers K, Mclellan AT, Jaeger JL, Pettinati HM. The development of the comprehensive addiction severity index for adolescents (Casi-A)—an interview for assessing multiple problems of adolescents. J Subst Abuse Treat. 1995;12:181–93.

Meyers K, Hagan TA, McDermott P, Webb A, Randall M, et al. Factor structure of the comprehensive adolescent severity inventory (CASI): results of reliability, validity, and generalizability analyses. Am J Drug Alcohol Abuse. 2006;32:287–310.

Moffitt T. Life-course-persistent versus adolescence-limited antisocial behaviour: a 10-year research review and a research agenda. In: Cicchetti D, Cohen DJ, editors. Developmental psychopathology, vol 3: risk, disorder, and adaptation. Hoboken, NJ: Wiley; 2006. p. 570–98.

Pullatz M, Bierman KL. Aggression, antisocial behaviour, and violence among girls: a developmental perspective. New York, NY: Guilford; 2004.

Reynolds CR, Kamphaus RW. Behavior assessment system for children. 2nd ed. Circle Pines, MN: American Guidance Service; 2004.

Scott S, Knapp M, Henderson J, Maughan B. Financial cost of social exclusion: follow up study of antisocial children into adulthood. BMJ. 2001;323(7306):191.

Straus MA, Hamby SL, BoneyMcCoy S, Sugarman DB. The revised conflict tactics scales (CTS2)—development and preliminary psychometric data. J Fam Issues. 1996;17:283–316.

The National Institute for Health and Care Excellence (NICE) (2013) guidelines.

ADHD and Substance Abuse in Children and Adolescents

7

7.1 Objectives

- Describe the prevalence and epidemiology of ADHD and Substance/Alcohol Use Disorder in adolescents and young adults
- Explain the Link Between ADHD and SUD
- List some of the psychiatric disorders that should be considered and included in the differential diagnosis when assessing individuals with substance use disorders
- Recognize some of the barriers to seeking Addiction treatment
- Describe tools and approaches that health professionals can use to screen for and diagnose substance use in adolescents.
- Describe some on the management considerations that clinicians should recognize when using ADHD medications in adolescents with ADHD and addictions
- List the principals of treatment for substance abusing adolescents with ADHD
- Describe the epidemiology, morbidity and common reasons for stimulant abuse and diversion

7.2 The Case

Read the following case and check if the clinician completed the following tasks in this case?

- Obtained full psychiatric and medical history?
- Used some rating scales or questionnaires during the assessment?
- Obtained collateral history?
- Reviewed functional impairment?
- Conducted appropriate investigations, blood work and physical exam as indicated?
- Documented the assessment?

J. Sadek, *Clinician's Guide to ADHD Comorbidities in Children and Adolescents*,
https://doi.org/10.1007/978-3-319-45635-5_7

- Reached a diagnosis and assessed for comorbid disorders?
- Communicated results of the assessment to the patient and family?
- Provided adequate education to patient and family?
- Explained the possible pharmacological and psychosocial treatments and alternatives?
- Provided appropriate management and treatment interventions
- Explained the risk and benefit of treatment and lack of treatment?
- Referred the patient to other services or resources in the community as indicated?
- Suggested appropriate accommodations?
- Provided a follow up appointment?

Shawn is a 17 year old boy in grade 11 who lives in Ottawa, Ontario with his father and his 15 year old brother. He was diagnosed with ADHD at age 8 but was never treated for ADHD because his father did not believe in ADHD treatment. Shawn's mother passed away in a car accident 3 years ago.

Chief Concern: Poor attendance record in school and poor academic performance. Father found Mushroom in the house.

History of present illness: Shawn said that he did not do well in school last year because of anxiety and acid reflux. He has always been anxious. He worries about his sport performance, and his father' health. His anxiety extends to everything and he cannot stop it since his mother passed away. He said: "I stress out about a lot of stuff and I put myself to high standard and I cannot do it".

He reported insomnia at times related to his anxiety. His appetite is good, tired all the time, mood is average and has no suicidal thoughts. He had suicidal thoughts after his mother's death but he is not having these dark thoughts anymore.

He gets panic attacks regularly. At times, he gets them before his basketball games.

In terms of ADHD Shawn and his father confirmed a long history that started in childhood and persisted in multiple settings of the following symptoms:

Fails to give close attention to details or makes careless mistakes in tasks

Has difficulty sustaining attention in tasks (few minutes)

Does not seem to listen when spoken to directly (frequent day dreaming)

Does not follow through on instructions and fails to finish school work, chores, or duties (persistent and frequent. Needs daily frequent reminders)

He is extremely disorganized in his home and school life.

Avoids, dislikes, or reluctantly engages in tasks requiring sustained mental effort (homework was a frequent struggle)

Loses things necessary for activities (mom could name many things)

Easily distracted by extraneous stimuli such as noise or movement.

Forgetful in daily activities (needs reminders)

Fidgets with hands or feet or squirms in seat (evident in the interview)

Runs about in situations in which it is inappropriate (instead of walking)

Had difficulty engaging in leisure activities quietly (as a child can get very loud).

Does things impulsively and without thinking

Interrupt others and has difficulty waiting his turn.

He states that school boring and he had a hard time concentrating on the material. He has a hard time holding down a summer job because he is always late and doesn't do the work properly. He reacts to slights violently and once assaulted a coworker who criticized him for being late. He describes himself as "a looser".

He did not want to discuss substance use in presence of his father so his father left the interview room. Shawn said he started drinking and smoking in grade 7 when he was 13 then started using Acid, Mushroom, weed, pain killers and clonazepam after the death of his mother.

Medical history: Has no known allergies. Has acid reflux.

Family history: Brother has anxiety. Father is a recovering alcoholic.

Personal history: There were no complications with mother's pregnancy.

The delivery was a vaginal delivery at term at the public hospital.

His birth weight was 7 pounds 3 ounces. There were no neonatal concerns and went home at 2 days of age. He was bottle fed and his immunizations were up-to-date.

Patient had neither gross nor fine motor problems.

No problems with milestones or social interactions.

He had small group of friends in elementary school but in high school started having lots of friends. Shawn is a good basketball player.

Case Outcome: Shawn was diagnosed with ADHD combined type, substance use disorder, Generalized anxiety disorder. His ADHD was treated successfully with atomoxetine and he started seeing psychologist for individual and family therapy. He continued to improve. Therapy started by motivational interviewing and continued with a CBT approach. Issues around grief were also addressed in therapy. Family therapy was very helpful since father was very supportive of Shawn.

7.3 Substance Use Literature Review Questions

7.3.1 Describe the Prevalence and Epidemiology of ADHD and Substance/Alcohol Use Disorder?

Comorbidity of Substance Use disorder and ADHD is high. Children with ADHD have been found to be at increased risk of developing SUDs (Zulauf et al. 2014; Groenman et al. 2017).

Substance use disorders are common in adolescents and adults with ADHD and some studies suggested that 33% of ADHD patients were having a history of an alcohol use disorder and 20% were having a drug use disorder (Kessler et al. 1996; Wilens et al. 2008a, b). Literature also suggests that one-quarter of adults with SUDs, and one-half of adolescents with SUDs, have ADHD. Adults with SUDs also show a higher risk for ADHD, as well as earlier onset, and more severe SUDs, associated with ADHD.

ADHD significantly increased the risk of for alcohol abuse, cannabis abuse, and other illicit substances, in both males and females, compared to individuals without ADHD (Ottosen et al. 2016).

The misuse of marijuana, alcohol, or the combination of the two are the most common substances of abuse in adolescents with ADHD but one important antecedent to developing SUD in children and adolescents with ADHD is cigarette smoking. Cocaine and stimulant abuse is not overrepresented in ADHD; but marijuana continues to be the most commonly abused agent (Wilens 2011; Wilens and Morrison 2011; Wilens et al. 2011).

7.3.2 Explain the Possible Link Between ADHD and SUD?

The self-medication hypothesis is plausible in ADHD. Moreover, the accompanying poor self-judgment and impulsivity associated with ADHD may be conducive to the development of SUD.

The second hypothesis relies on neurobiological link. Functional imaging studies have demonstrated that there may be deficits in anterior cingulate activation and the frontosubcortical systems, dompaminergic transmission and reward system in both individuals with ADHD and SUD (Cortese et al. 2013).

Genetic and family research support the link between ADHD and SUD. It appears that exposure to nicotine, alcohol or substances during pregnancy increases the risk of development of ADHD in the offspring. Literature also has shown that siblings, parents, and offspring of individuals with SUD share the etiologies of ADHD and SUD as well as several genes.

Comorbid disorders may also support the link between ADHD and SUD. Co-occurring conduct or bipolar disorders increase risk of SUD among ADHD patients.

Some controversy exists about the relationship between ADHD treatment and substance use. (Zulauf et al. 2014). Some researchers suggest that there is not enough evidence to support an increase or reduction of SUD risk associated with ADHD medication (Humphreys et al. 2013).

Others suggest that ADHD treatment reduce later substance use disorders in adolescence (Wilens et al. 2003; Groenman et al. 2013; Hammerness et al. 2013; Molina et al. 2013).

7.3.3 Describe Some of the Challenges in the Diagnostic Assessment of ADHD and SUD?

Substance effects during acute intoxication or withdrawal may produce overlapping symptoms with ADHD such as impulsivity, agitation, mood instability, intolerance to frustrations, restlessness, concentration and memory difficulties.

Craving and loss of control which are common part of the addictive process may also overlap with ADHD with symptoms of Impulsivity, poor decision making, planning difficulties, mood instability and continued substance use in spite of adverse consequences.

Deficits in Executive function may be pre-existing in both patients of ADHD and SUD with symptoms of impulsivity, risk-taking behavior, inattention and inability to inhibit responses.

Common psychiatric comorbidities to addictions such as mood and anxiety disorders, borderline and antisocial personality disorder may produce symptoms depression, anxiety may show several overlapping symptoms of ADHD such as impulsivity, risk-taking behavior and intolerance to frustration (Fatseas et al. 2012).

7.3.4 What Psychiatric Disorders Should Be Considered and Included in the Differential Diagnosis When Assessing Individuals with Substance Use Disorders?

Mood disorders (both unipolar depression and bipolar disorder), anxiety disorders, ADHD, personality disorders (Borderline and antisocial), effect of substance (withdrawal, intoxication), sleep disorders such as obstructive sleep apnea, endocrine and metabolic disorders such as thyroid disorders, neurological disorders (traumatic brain injury) (Zulauf et al. 2014).

7.3.5 What Are Some of the Barriers to Seeking Addiction Treatment?

Major Barriers to Addiction Treatment include:

- Stigma: perhaps one of the largest obstacle. In society, there is significant shame and stigma around addiction issues, where it remains viewed by many as a moral failing or lack of self-control. As a result, people are very hesitant to seek appropriate treatment, or do so in secrecy which is often unhelpful as it exacerbates the shame and increases the risk of relapse.
- Lack of appropriate resources - particularly in rural areas, there may be very limited treatment options. Larger areas have more resources, but may not be easily accessible.
- Unrecognized or untreated mental illness: psychosis, anxiety, depression or other mental health issues may prevent patients from seeking treatment, as they attempt to "self-medicate" their psychological symptoms with mood altering substances. Similarly, if they do seek treatment for addiction issues and these co-morbid conditions are not addressed, this dramatically worsens their prognosis and increases the risk of relapse.
- Primary support network that also use or abuse substances: many people find that those close to them in fact enable their ongoing substance use, and find it difficult to create a new support network of those who are supportive of positive change in their lives.
- Cost of treatment for patients who have limited income or unable to access public resources
- Fear of consequences particularly if here there are concerns that addiction treatment may be used against them in some manner.

- Ethnicity, culture and gender specific issues: In some areas in the United States and Canada, the majority of those who seek treatment are Caucasian. Some cultural issues might also contribute to help seeking behaviour. Gender specific issues particularly for women have been widely discussed in the literature.
- Lack of insight: many patients with addictions do not acknowledge that there is a problem so they do not seek help. Motivation enhancement techniques can be very helpful in these situations. Motivational Interview is a method for enhancing motivation by exploring and resolving ambivalence. The principles of motivational interviewing include: asking open-ended questions, providing patient affirmation, practicing reflective listening, and summarizing (Probst et al. 2015; Saunders et al. 2006).

7.3.6 What Models of Care Are Used to Treat Concurrent Disorders in Patients with Substance Abuse? What Are the Strengths and Weaknesses of These Models?

Three primary models of service delivery exist for concurrent disorders:

1. Sequential Treatment

   In sequential treatment, the individual seeks treatment for one disorder. Then—having successfully addressed that disorder—the patient moves on to treatment for the second disorder. The more serious or severe condition, viewed as the primary disorder, is generally tackled first. This approach may delay much-needed interventions.

   Most often, a person's two conditions are interrelated, so it can be very difficult to address the issues in isolation from one another. For example, addressing a drinking problem in someone who is profoundly depressed presents a serious clinical challenge. Often, sequential treatment results in neither condition receiving adequate or timely treatment. In this type of sequential approach, patients often end up going from one service to the other repeatedly, a frustrating experience that can cause them to give up on treatment entirely.
2. Parallel Treatment

   In this model, individuals are cared for with a coordinated clinical care approach, one which addresses both mental health issues and addictions concerns together, drawing on the strengths and expertise of both types of clinical approaches. Mental health issues are tackled by those on the mental health team. At the same time, substance use issues are addressed by addictions staff. This type of treatment helps improve the individual's likelihood of successful recovery. The challenge to success in this model, however, is effective communication between caregivers. With multiple professionals involved, an accountability system is needed to ensure that clinicians communicate regularly with one another and not give conflicting advice or messages to patients based on differing treatment practices and philosophies.

3. Integrated Treatment

In this model, patients receive treatment for all their addiction and mental health conditions under the care of a single multidisciplinary team. The theory behind this treatment model is that one cohesive team simultaneously addressing all aspects of mental health and addictions may improve outcomes (Torrens et al. 2012).

7.3.7 Suggest a Screening Tool for Adolescent Substance/Alcohol Use Disorder?

CRAFT questionnaire: Brief screening for adolescents with substance use.

Screening using the CRAFFT begins by asking the adolescent to "Please answer these next questions honestly"; telling him/her "Your answers will be kept confidential"; and then asking three opening questions.

C—Have you ever ridden in a **C**AR driven by someone (including yourself) who was "high" or who had been using alcohol or drugs?

R—Do you ever use alcohol or drugs to **R**ELAX, feel better about yourself, or fit in?

A—Do you ever use alcohol or drugs while you are **A**LONE?

F—Do you ever **F**ORGET things you did while using alcohol or drugs?

F—Do your family or **F**RIENDS ever tell you that you should cut down on your drinking or drug use?

T—Have you gotten into **T**ROUBLE while you were using alcohol or drugs?

Two or more yes answers suggest a significant problem. The CRAFFT questions. http://www.ceasar-boston.org/CRAFFT/

7.3.8 What Are the National Institute of Drug Abuse Principals of Treatment of Substance Use Disorders in Adolescents?

- Adolescent substance use needs to be identified and addressed as soon as possible.
- Adolescents can benefit from a drug abuse intervention even if they are not addicted to a drug.
- Routine annual medical visits are an opportunity to ask adolescents about drug use.
- Legal interventions and sanctions or family pressure may play an important role in getting adolescents to enter, stay in, and complete treatment.
- Substance use disorder treatment should be tailored to the unique needs of the adolescent.
- Treatment should address the needs of the whole person, rather than just focusing on his or her drug use.
- Behavioral therapies are effective in addressing adolescent drug use.

- Families and the community are important aspects of treatment
- Effectively treating substance use disorders in adolescents requires also identifying and treating any other mental health conditions they may have
- Sensitive issues such as violence and child abuse or risk of suicide should be identified and addressed.
- It is important to monitor drug use during treatment.
- Staying in treatment for an adequate period of time and continuity of care afterward are important.
- Testing adolescents for sexually transmitted diseases like HIV, as well as hepatitis B and C, is an important part of drug treatment (**www.drugabuse.gov**)

7.3.9 Describe Some on the Controversial Management Considerations That Clinicians Face When Using ADHD Medications in Individuals with ADHD and Addictions?

ADHD medications appear to have little to no efficacy in the treatment of co-morbid addictive disorders but do not appear to exacerbate addictive disorders. Majority of the controlled clinical trials did not find enough evidence of exacerbation but it should be noted that a few cases of abuse and misuse have been reported in uncontrolled clinical studies.

ADHD medications appear less effective in ADHD patients with addictive disorders compared to patients without these co-morbid disorders. It appears that although the various medications (both stimulants and non-stimulants) assessed in several studies can improve ADHD in the short term, they are less effective in ADHD patients with addictive disorders than in patients without these co-morbid disorders. Researchers challenge the available evidence and consider it ambiguous in terms of whether differences in adherence affect clinical outcomes in patients treated for ADHD.

ADHD medications seem to exert a strong placebo effect on ADHD symptoms in patients with addictive disorders. Some studies report placebo response rates as high as 45–55% in adults. The high placebo response may be related to a non-specific effect of addiction treatment on impulsivity and aggressiveness. Such an effect probably lessens the severity of some clinical manifestations of ADHD. Another possible explanation may be related to the high expectations of patients with addictions or their treating clinicians that medical treatment will improve ADHD symptoms.

Possibly the concomitant psychosocial treatment (mainly cognitive behavioral therapy) in many of the controlled studies may have contributed to the reported efficacy of the ADHD medications.

Some researchers suggest that ADHD and SUD-related craving share neurobiological similarities, and that treatment of ADHD may reduce craving for substances and subsequently reduce the risk for relapse to substance use. An aggregate of the literature seems to suggest that early stimulant treatment reduces, or delays, the onset of SUDs and perhaps cigarette smoking into adolescence; however, the protective effect is lost in adulthood. These issues remain unclear and further research is needed in these areas.

7.3.10 Describe Some of the Factors That Help Make the Decision of How Long to Wait for SUD to Be Under Control Before Initiating Pharmacological Treatment of ADHD

The relationship between ADHD and SUD is bidirectional. The decision to treat or not treat ADHD in the context of active substance abuse depends on numerous factors. Among these are:

1. The type and severity of substance involved.
2. The patient's opinion about the importance of ADHD in his/her particular case.
3. The degree of diagnostic uncertainty for ADHD.
4. The risk of exacerbating SUD and other mental disorders by treating ADHD.
5. The experience of the treatment team in the management of SUD and ADHD co-morbidity,
6. The ability to closely monitor the patient's adherence and response to treatment.

It is recommended to individualize the treatment decision due to the multiple challenges of ADHD and SUD comorbidity. The decision should be done on a case-by-case basis in which the arguments for and against immediate pharmacological treatment of ADHD are carefully weighed. The results of such an assessment will indicate when to initiate ADHD treatment and the most appropriate choice of medication.

7.3.11 Is There an Association Between Stimulant Medication and Substance Use Disorder?

Stimulant medications not only lower concurrent risk but also lower long-term risk of substance-related events. ADHD medication is unlikely to be associated with greater risk of substance-related problems in adolescence or adulthood (Quinn et al. 2017).

Patients who initiated treatment of ADHD at an early age (aged 9 or younger) had lower risk for substance use compared to those who initiated treatment in adolescence (McCabe et al. 2016).

Longer duration of stimulant medication therapy for ADHD was associated with lower rates of substance use during late adolescence as compared to shorter duration of stimulant medication therapy for ADHD at all developmental periods, especially among those who initiated stimulant medication therapy for ADHD in preschool, elementary, and middle school. However, the length of duration of stimulant medication therapy for ADHD on substance use appeared to play a less pronounced role among those who initiated stimulant medication therapy for ADHD in high school (McCabe et al. 2016).

7.3.12 What Are the Unique Needs of Adolescents with Substance Use Disorders?

- Adolescent drug abusers have unique needs stemming from their immature neurocognitive and psychosocial stage of development. Research suggests that the brain areas most closely associated with aspects of behavior such as decision-making, judgment, planning, and self-control undergo a period of rapid development during adolescence and young adulthood therefore adolescents need additional support during that period.
- Adolescent drug abuse is also often comorbid with ADHD, ODD, conduct disorder, mood and anxiety disorders. Treatment of comorbid disorders are very valuable.
- Positive family involvement into the care of adolescents as well as integrating other systems in which the adolescent participates in such as school and athletics, and recognize the importance of prosocial peer relationships are very important in effective treatment because adolescents are very sensitive to social cues.
- Medications for substance abuse among adolescents may in certain cases be helpful (NIDA 2012).

7.3.13 What Are the Treatment Recommendations for Substance Abusing Patients with ADHD?

The strategy for caring for patients with SUD and ADHD should include consideration of both disorders. A complete assessment of the substance use and ADHD needs be conducted prior to treatment. Once the substance use is better controlled or in a harm reduction model, the uses of psychotherapeutic intervention such as motivational interviewing, family therapy and CBT appear to be useful as a first step for addressing both the ADHD and SUD. They would incorporate structured and goal-directed sessions as well as active therapist involvement. Additionally, pharmacological agents can be used in conjunction with psychotherapy in order to alleviate ADHD symptoms and further substance use. Psycho-education is also useful. Furthermore, young adults with SUD benefit from both family and individual intervention.

Several review studies have suggested that the use of nonstimulant agents (atomoxetine), extended-release or longer acting stimulants with lower abuse liability and diversion and potential antidepressants (bupropion) is preferable when treating patients with comorbid ADHD and SUD (Knecht et al. 2015; American family physician).

There have been some differences in the literature regarding response to atomoxetine depending upon the time the treatment was initiated (e.g., whether the study subjects were actively engaging in substance abuse or dependence versus being engaged in brief abstinence). Further research is also needed in these areas (Zulauf et al. 2014).

Psychotherapeutic interventions in addition to pharmacological treatment can be beneficial. Cognitive behavioral therapy (CBT) may be of particular interest, and neurofeeedback (given preliminary evidence suggesting its possible efficacy in adolescents with comorbid ADHD and SUD (Thurstone et al. 2010).

The Family Therapy models most commonly noted in the research literature for adolescent substance use include Brief Strategic Family Therapy (BSFT), Family Behavior Therapy, Functional Family Therapy (FFT), Multidimensional Family Therapy (MDFT), and Multisystem Family Therapy (MST).

Adolescent Community Reinforcement Approach (A-CRA) is designed to increase adolescents' access to reinforce through operant conditioning principles and skills-training activities so that non–substance-using behaviors are rewarded and can replace substance use behavior. It includes a combination of CBT (with an emphasis on behavioral procedures) and caregiver/family procedures. It uses a positive, non-confrontational approach to promote abstinence, healthy social activities, positive peer relationships, and improved relationships with family. It has been successfully used for ADHD and SUD comorbidity in adolescents (Godley et al. 2014).

7.3.14 Suggest Some Web Resources for Adolescents with Substance Use Disorder?

National Institute on Drug Abuse.

Web site: http://www.nida.nih.gov/students.html

SAMHSA's National Clearing House for Alcohol and Drug Information:

Tips for Teens Free alcohol and drug informational brochures.

Web site: http://ncadistore.samhsa.gov/catalog/pubseries.aspx

SAMHSA's National Mental Health Information Center.

Comprehensive information on children's mental health, hotlines, and links to other useful sites.

Web site: http://mentalhealth.samhsa.gov

7.3.15 Describe Some of the Concepts Related to Stimulant Medications Abuse and Misuse?

Stimulant medications, like illicit psychostimulants, have the potential to induce abuse and dependence. Along with opioids and central nervous system depressants, stimulants are one of the most commonly abused pharmaceutical drug classes.

Some evidence for the abuse liability of pharmaceutical stimulants can be found in both animal and human Research. Stimulant-induced elevations in brain dopamine appear to be integral to both efficacy in ADHD and potential for abuse (Clemow and Walker 2014).

These stimulant medications, particularly when injected or in immediate-release form, could produce subjective and reinforcing effects similar to the illicit psychostimulants. Some researchers argued that much of the concern about these medications is based on reports of 'misuse', rather than 'abuse'. Misuse can range from non-compliance to compulsive abuse (Kollins 2008).

7.3.16 What Is the Rate of Stimulants Misuse or Abuse in Young People?

About one in every six US adolescents has ever used prescription stimulants either medically or non-medically (McCabe and West 2013).

The National Institute of Drug Abuse (NIDA)'s monitoring the future survey of substance use and attitudes in teens in the US found that about 1 in 13 high school seniors reported past-year nonmedical use of the prescription stimulant Adderall® in 2015 (The University of Michigan Institute for Social Research 2016).

Estimate of 21.3% of US high school seniors reported lifetime medical or non-medical use of prescription stimulants by age 18 years (1976–1996) and 13.1% reported nonmedical use of prescription stimulants only (with no history of medical use) (McCabe et al. 2017).

Among US and Canadian school students, the reported prevalence of past-year pharmaceutical stimulant misuse is 5–9%. Studies of stimulant misuse among university/college students have yielded life-time prevalence estimates of 7–17%, and 5–35% for past-year.

One recent studies of misuse have found life-time prevalence rates of 5–43% and past-year prevalence rates of 5–6%.

Misuse peak prevalence from 16 to 24 years of age, with a decline over subsequent years. Stimulant medications misuse or abuse is more prevalent on university/college campuses than among young adults in the general population. In one study, students aged 18–22 years were more than twice as likely to report misuse of MPH in the past year (6.4% versus 3.0%). Mixed amphetamine salts were more likely to have been misused among college students than non-student peers (7.9% versus 5.4%) (Kollins 2008; Clemow and Walker 2014).

7.3.17 What Are the Correlates of Diversion and Misuse?

1. Higher rates of hyperactivity–impulsivity
2. Conduct disorder
3. Other illicit drug use
4. Male
5. Caucasian
6. A college or university attendee (Clemow and Walker 2014)

7.3.18 Describe Some of the Research Findings on Stimulant Medications Diversion?

There are few studies that have reported specifically on diversion. Research (Wilens et al. 2011) found reports of diversion in six of the studies they reviewed, with life-time rates of diversion ranging from 11 to 29%. Personal experience of diversion appears far less prevalent than knowledge of diversion among others. Sharp & Rosen found that, while only 8%of students had sold or given away medication themselves, 63% knew someone else who had done so, and 67% knew someone who had taken stimulant medication recreationally. Other studies have measured the prevalence of students with prescriptions being asked to sell, trade or give away their medication, with 23–84% of students having been approached (Wilens et al. 2011; Rabiner 2013).

7.3.19 What Are the Reasons of Abuse or Misuse of Stimulant Medications?

1. To improve attention, concentration and alertness, study habits and academic performance
2. Pleasure seeking and to get high
3. Craving
4. Habits or Impulsivity (Newton 2009; Rabiner 2013)

7.3.20 What Are the Clinical Implications of Stimulants Abuse or Diversion?

Those diverting ADHD medication are not receiving the full benefits of pharmacotherapy and those receiving diverted medication are placing themselves at unnecessary risk of adverse health effects or toxicity (Rabiner 2013).

Recent research suggests that adolescent nonmedical users of prescription stimulants (with or without medical use) had lower educational attainment and more SUD symptoms in adulthood, compared to population controls and medical users of prescription stimulants without nonmedical use during adolescence (McCabe et al. 2017).

Withdrawal symptoms associated with discontinuing stimulant use include fatigue, depression, and disturbed sleep patterns. Repeated misuse of some stimulants (sometimes within a short period) can lead to serious adverse effects in addition to feelings of hostility or paranoia, or even psychosis (Hart and Ksir 2013).

References

Clemow DB, Walker DJ. The potential for misuse and abuse of medications in ADHD: a review. Postgrad Med. 2014;126(5):64–81. https://doi.org/10.3810/pgm.2014.09.2801. Review. PubMed PMID: 25295651

Cortese S, Holtmann M, Banaschewski T, et al. Practitioner review: current best practice in the management of adverse events during treatment with ADHD medications in children and adolescents. J Child Psychol Psychiatry. 2013;54:227–46.

Fatseas M, Debrabant R, Auriacombe M. The diagnostic accuracy of attention-deficit/hyperactivity disorder in adults with substance use disorders. Curr Opin Psychiatry. 2012;25(3):219–25.

Godley SH, Smith JE, Passetti LL, Subramaniam G. The Adolescent Community Reinforcement Approach (A-CRA) as a model paradigm for the management of adolescents with substance use disorders and co-occurring psychiatric disorders. Subst Abus. 2014;35(4):352–63.

Groenman AP, Oosterlaan J, Rommelse NN, et al. Stimulant treatment for attention-deficit hyperactivity disorder and risk of developing substance use disorder. Br J Psychiatry. 2013;203:112–9.

Groenman AP, Janssen TWP, Oosterlaan J. Childhood psychiatric disorders as risk factor for subsequent substance abuse: a meta-analysis. J Am Acad Child Adolesc Psychiatry. 2017;56(7):556–69.

Hammerness P, Joshi G, Doyle R, et al. Do stimulants reduce the risk for cigarette smoking in youth with attention-deficit hyperactivity disorder? A prospective, long-term, open-label study of extended-release methylphenidate. J Pediatr 2013;162:22–27e2.

Hart CL, Ksir C. Drugs, society & human behavior. 15th ed. New York, NY: McGraw-Hill; 2013.

Humphreys KL, Eng T, Lee SS. Stimulant medication and substance use outcomes: a meta-analysis. JAMA Psychiat. 2013;70:740–9.

Kessler RC, Nelson CB, McGonagle KA, Edlund MJ, Frank RG, Leaf PJ. The epidemiology of co-occurring addictive and mental disorders: implications for prevention and service utilization. Am J Orthopsychiatry. 1996;66(1):17–31.PubMed PMID: 8720638.

Knecht C, de Alvaro R, Martinez-Raga J, Balanza-Martinez V. Attention-deficit hyperactivity disorder (ADHD), substance use disorders, and criminality: a difficult problem with complex solutions. Int J Adolesc Med Health. 2015;27(2):163–75.

Kollins SH. A qualitative review of issues arising in the use of psycho-stimulant medications in patients with ADHD and co-morbid substance use disorders. Curr Med Res Opin. 2008;24(5):1345–57.

McCabe SE, West BT. Medical and nonmedical use of prescription stimulants: results from a national multicohort study. J Am Acad Child Adolesc Psychiatry. 2013;52(12):1272–80.

McCabe SE, Dickinson K, West BT, Wilens TE. Age of onset, duration, and type of medication therapy for attention-deficit/hyperactivity disorder and substance use during adolescence: a multi-cohort national study. J Am Acad Child Adolesc Psychiatry. 2016;55(6):479–86.

McCabe SE, Veliz P, Wilens TE, Schulenberg JE. Adolescents' prescription stimulant use and adult functional outcomes: a national prospective study. J Am Acad Child Adolesc Psychiatry. 2017;56(3):226–233.e4.

Molina BS, Hinshaw SP, Eugene AL, et al. Adolescent substance use in the multimodal treatment study of attention-deficit/hyperactivity disorder (ADHD) (MTA) as a function of childhood ADHD, random assignment to childhood treatments, and subsequent medication. J Am Acad Child Adolesc Psychiatry. 2013;52:250–63.

Newton TF. Theories of addiction: methamphetamine users' explanations for continuing drug use and relapse. Am J Add. 2009;18(4):294–300.

NIDA. Principles of drug addiction treatment: a research-based guide. 3rd ed. December 2012. https://d14rmgtrwzf5a.cloudfront.net/sites/default/files/podat_1.pdf

Ottosen C, Petersen L, Larsen JT, Dalsgaard S. Gender differences in associations between attention-deficit/hyperactivity disorder and substance use disorder. J Am Acad Child Adolesc Psychiatry. 2016;55(3):227–234.e4.

Probst C, Manthey J, Martinez A, Rehm J. Alcohol use disorder severity and reported reasons not to seek treatment: a cross-sectional study in European primary care practices. Subst Abuse Treat Prev Policy. 2015;10:32.

Quinn PD, Chang Z, Hur K, Gibbons RD, Lahey BB, Rickert ME, Sjölander A, Lichtenstein P, Larsson H, D'Onofrio BM. ADHD medication and substance-related problems. Am J Psychiatry. 2017;174(9):877–85.

Rabiner DL. Stimulant prescription cautions: addressing misuse, diversion and malingering. Curr Psychiatry Rep. 2013;15(7):375. https://doi.org/10.1007/s11920-013-0375-2. Review. PubMed PMID: 23712725

Saunders SM, Zygowicz KM, D'Angelo BR. Person-related and treatment-related barriers to alcohol treatment. J Subst Abus Treat. 2006;30(3):261–70.

The University of Michigan Institute for Social Research. Monitoring the future national survey results on drug use, 1975–2015: overview, key findings on adolescent drug use February 2016.

Thurstone C, Riggs PD, Salomonsen-Sautel S, Mikulich-Gilbertson SK. Randomized, controlled trial of atomoxetine for attention-deficit/hyperactivity disorder in adolescents with substance use disorder. J Am Acad Child Adolesc Psychiatry. 2010;49(6):573–82.

Torrens M, Rossi PC, Martinez-Riera R, Martinez-Sanvisens D, Bulbena A. Psychiatric comorbidity and substance use disorders: treatment in parallel systems or in one integrated system? Subst Use Misuse. 2012;47(8–9):1005–14.

Wilens T, et al. Does stimulant therapy of ADHD beget later substance abuse: a metanalytic review of the literature. Pediatrics. 2003;11(1):179–85.

Wilens TE, Adamson J, Monuteaux MC, Faraone SV, Schillinger M, Westerberg D, Biederman J. Effect of prior stimulant treatment for attention-deficit/hyperactivity disorder on subsequent risk for cigarette smoking and alcohol and drug use disorders in adolescents. Arch Pediatr Adolesc Med. 2008a;162(10):916–21. https://doi.org/10.1001/archpedi.162.10.916. PubMed PMID: 18838643;PubMed Central PMCID: PMC2760975.

Wilens TE, Adler LA, Adams J, Sgambati S, Rotrosen J, Sawtelle R, Utzinger L, Fusillo S. Misuse and diversion of stimulants prescribed for ADHD: a systematic review of the literature. J Am Acad Child Adolesc Psychiatry. 2008b;47(1):21–31. https://doi.org/10.1097/chi.0b013e31815a56f1. Review. PubMed PMID:18174822.

Wilens TE. A sobering fact: ADHD leads to substance abuse. J Am Acad Child Adolesc Psychiatry. 2011;50(1):6–8. https://doi.org/10.1016/j.jaac.2010.10.002.

Wilens TE, Morrison NR. The intersection of attention-deficit/hyperactivity disorder and substance abuse. Curr Opin Psychiatry. 2011;24(4):280–5. https://doi.org/10.1097/YCO.0b013e328345c956.

Wilens TE, Martelon M, Joshi G, Bateman C, Fried R, Petty C, Biederman J. Does ADHD predict substance-use disorders? A 10-year follow-up study of young adults with ADHD. J Am Acad Child Adolesc Psychiatry. 2011;50(6):543–53. https://doi.org/10.1016/j.

Zulauf CA, Sprich SE, Safren SA, et al. The complicated relationship between attention deficit/hyperactivity disorder and substance use disorders. Curr Psychiatry Rep. 2014;16:436.

8 ADHD and Specific Learning Disorders

8.1 Objectives

- Describe the rates of comorbidities between ADHD and Specific learning Disorders
- Describe the possible risk factors of ADHD and specific Learning disorders
- Describe the diagnostic and management approaches of ADHD and SLD

8.2 Case Vignette

Read the following case and check if the clinician completed the following tasks in this case?

- Obtained full psychiatric and medical history?
- Used some rating scales or questionnaires during the assessment?
- Obtained collateral history?
- Reviewed functional impairment?
- Conducted appropriate investigations, blood work and physical exam as indicated?
- Documented the assessment?
- Reached a diagnosis and assessed for comorbid disorders?
- Communicated results of the assessment to the patient and family?
- Provided adequate education to patient and family?
- Explained the possible pharmacological and psychosocial treatments and alternatives?
- Provided appropriate management and treatment interventions
- Explained the risk and benefit of treatment and lack of treatment?
- Referred the patient to other services or resources in the community as indicated?
- Suggested appropriate accommodations?
- Provided a follow up appointment?

J. Sadek, *Clinician's Guide to ADHD Comorbidities in Children and Adolescents*,
https://doi.org/10.1007/978-3-319-45635-5_8

Lena Long is an 8 year old girl who lives in Ottawa with her 12 year old brother and her mother.

Mom and grandmother came to the interview. Mom said that her child complains that her brain is not working right and that she is having so many problems in school. She is unable to read despite lots of support from teachers and having a tutor after school.

Medically she is healthy. Weight is 27 kg and heights 125 cm

Mother was diabetic and had grave's disease during the pregnancy. Delivery was induced and Lena was purple at Birth. No fine or gross motor problems. She had delayed speech but no hearing problems.

School reported that Lena does not finish her school work, she disrupts the class, day dream and does not listen when teachers are talking to her. She does not stop talking and leaves her seat frequently. Teachers mentioned that she cannot read appropriately and does not understand what she reads.

Her Brother has ADHD and treated Methylphenidate.

Her father was out of the picture since she was 5 month old but her grandfather is very involved in her care.

Mother mentioned that she was diagnosed with ADHD combined type by her pediatrician 2 years ago but family refused treatment.

8.3 Review Questions

8.3.1 What Are the Rates of Comorbidities Between ADHD and Specific Learning Disorders?

Specific learning Disorders fall under three broad sub-categories: Reading disorders (RDS), written language disorder (WLD), and mathematics disorder (MD). They have high comorbidity with ADHD ranging from 31 to 45% (DuPaul et al. 2013; Pennington 2006).

Reading Disorders (RDs) account for approximately 80% of all specific learning disorders (SLDs) and has a comorbidity rate with ADHD between 25 and 48%. In particular, dyslexia, a subset of RD involving difficulties with word recognition and decoding, is highly comorbid with ADHD, with 25–40% co-occurrence rate (Pham and Riviere 2015).

Mathematics disorder (MD) comorbidity rate with ADHD is estimated to be 11–30% (Capano et al. 2008).

Written language disorder (WLD) comorbidity rate with ADHD is estimated to be 55–64% (Pham and Riviere 2015).

8.3.2 Discuss the Possible Risk Factors of ADHD and Specific Learning Disorders?

Children with reading disorders (RDs) and ADHD alone Children with comorbid RD and ADHD often have a stronger genetic loading for both disorders and display a more severe profile of neuropsychological deficits and outcomes when compared to children with reading disorders (RDS) alone (Boada et al. 2012).

The high rate of comorbidity between ADHD and SLD suggest that the presence of either SLD or ADHD increases an individual's risks of developing the other disorder (Dupaul et al. 2013).

Reading Disorders and ADHD may have shared factors in neuropsychological profile related to processing speed, working memory and inattention (Boada et al. 2012; Rosenberg et al. 2012; Pham and Hasson 2014).

Some researchers found a reciprocal relationship between processing speed, rapid automatized naming (RAN), and inattention, all of which are found deficient in many children with ADHD (Arnett et al. 2012).

Research exploring the neuropsychological profile of Mathematics disorder (MD) and ADHD is limited. Children with MDs generally demonstrate weaknesses in either calculation or mathematical problem-solving and reasoning. Deficit in visuospatial or numerical working memory and processing speed may be related to failure with automatization (i.e., retrieval of basic math facts) and may be part of the neuropsychological profile of both disorders (Semrud-Clikeman and Bledsoe 2011). Others suggested that inattention is more closely related to mathematical skill deficits (Faraone et al. 2005).

Children with ADHD are also at an increased risk of exhibiting difficulties with written expression. In particular, children with often demonstrate weaknesses in visual-motor integration and fine motor coordination, which are often observed in ADHD (Pitcher et al. 2003; Pham and Riviere 2015).

ADHD related difficulties in various cognitive processes such as attention, working memory, organization, and planning can also affect the writing process (Yoshimasu et al. 2011)

Handwriting quality, spelling, and written expression are impaired in children with ADHD, compared to others without ADHD (Re et al. 2007).

Researchers suggest exploring the functioning of children who demonstrate deficits in technical aspects of writing (e.g., spelling, punctuation, grammar, etc.) and those with fine motor difficulties associated with writing (e.g., handwriting). They also suggest the need for additional studies to examine cognitive profiles among children with MD, particularly as it relates to processing speed and working memory in both domains (Pham and Riviere 2015). There is also strong genetic predisposition to both ADHD and SLD.

8.3.3 Discuss the Complexity in the Assessment and Diagnosis of SLD?

Assessments are crucial for understanding a child's abilities in order to tailor teaching content to specific needs, and for measuring progress over time to determine whether the teaching program is effective.

Assessments must measure the skills that aim to improve via the intervention, such as word reading accuracy or reading comprehension, and the foundational subskills that can be used in training (e.g., phoneme awareness or listening comprehension, respectively). The assessment also must include reliable and sensitive tests of these skills (Duff and Clarke 2011).

Some of the tests used in the assessment of specific learning disorders include Woodcock Reading Mastery Tests from age 5 years and older to assess Individual strengths and weaknesses in reading skills.

Comprehensive Test of Phonological Processing is used from age 5 to 24 years to test Phonologic awareness, phonologic memory, rapid naming, rhyming words, and decoding skills.

The KeyMath-3 Diagnostic Assessment is a widely used assessment of children's mathematical abilities (Kim et al. 2015).

Woodcock-Johnson Tests of Achievement-third edition (WJ II-Achv) is designed to measure both academic achievements and cognitive abilities for children, adolescents and adults.

DSM-IV diagnosis of LD relied was determined if a child's performance on standardized achievement tests is substantially below (more than 2 standard deviations (SDs) between achievement and IQ or 1–2 SDs if comorbid factors are present) expectations based on age, schooling, and intelligence level (APA 2000). However, changes were needed for many reasons including the limitations and errors in measurement of IQ and achievement tests that make the reliability and validity of that method questionable (Pham and Riviere 2015).

Currently in DSM-V, Specific learning Disorder (SLD) is now part of the neurodevelopmental disorders and requires 6 month or more of multiple sub-skill impairments individuals may demonstrate in various academic domains (e.g., reading, mathematics, written expressions).

Each area has to be specified according the following:

Reading Disorders should be specified into:

Word reading accuracy (which may include decoding),

Reading fluency,

Reading comprehension.

Impairments in mathematics should be specified into:

Number sense

Calculation accuracy

Memorization of arithmetic facts

Accurate math reasoning

Impairment in written expression were also delineated the following areas:

Spelling accuracy

Grammar and punctuation accuracy

Clarity or organization of written expressions

The age of onset has also been clarified by specifying that the difficulties may not be manifested until later when academic demands become more intense.

Children or adolescents with SLD often underachieve in multiple academic domains and often with pervasive negative consequences.

In addition, academic skills as evidenced by low achievement scores on norm-referenced standardized tests are required to be below (e.g., 1.5 SD) the individual's chronological age/grade level or on criterion-referenced tests that reveal average academic performance can only be sustained by tremendous effort, support, and services.

There are criteria of exclusion that exclude the diagnosis such as medical, psychiatric, language or lack of instruction.

8.3.4 What Are the Management Approaches of ADHD and SLD?

Multimodal treatment strategies are suggested for management of ADHD and SLD.

Researchers suggested that early recognition of reading disorders in children and early effective intervention in preschool or first grade are important to achieving good outcomes (Compton et al. 2006; Vellutino et al. 2006).

Clinicians should rule out secondary causes for both disorders and whether there is any evidence for a biologically treatable neurological disorder such as epilepsy or a genetic, metabolic, or structural brain disorder that might mandate EEG, brain imaging, or other investigations. Clinicians should determine that Learning difficulties are primarily not due to the following reasons: Lack of instruction in math, reading or writing, a visual, hearing or motor disability, Intellectual Disability, Emotional Disturbance, Cultural factors, Environmental or economic disadvantage or Limited language proficiency.

Treatment of comorbid disorders such as anxiety, or depression amenable to counseling and pharmacologic interventions, and for unfavorable environmental circumstances to be addressed. Dealing with these nonspecific issues together with cognitive counseling may determine the success or failure of remedial educational interventions (Rapin 2016).

Reading disorders may respond to specific interventions. Phonological-based interventions are generally effective in improving word reading in children with dyslexic difficulties. These interventions typically comprise training in phoneme awareness, letter knowledge, explicit and systematic instruction in phonics, and the application of these skills to the tasks of reading and writing (Duff and Clarke 2011).

PHAST (phonological and strategy training), is a program that has empiric support for improving phonemic awareness and basic reading skills. It combines training in phonological analysis, word blending, and word identification strategy, as well as a program developed to increase reading fluency in decoding and comprehension (Retrieval, Automaticity, Vocabulary elaboration, and Enrichment with language Orthography [RAVE-O]) Fletcher et al., 2005. The Peer-Assisted Learning Strategies (PALS) also has been shown to improve phonemic awareness and coding (Fuchs and Fuchs 2005).

Improvement of reading comprehension also has been studied, with emphasis on direct teaching of planning, prioritizing, organizing, and flexibility to enhance comprehension (Melzer et al. 2007). Computers also have been used that incorporate a speech synthesizer that can read the words that the child does not know (i.e., DECtalk) (Olson and Wise 2006).

Similarly, a computer program that highlights text while simultaneously reading the words has been found to improve spontaneous word recall and reading comprehension in children with RDs, ADHD, and emotional disturbance (Steele et al. 1996).

Mathematic learning disorders may benefit from specific interventions. Some studies have found improvement in a specific area of mathematics performance when students are provided with performance feedback and are also provided with explicit teaching of mathematics concepts and processes (Baker et al. 2002).

Some researchers suggested that math problem solving improve when teacher instruction of mathematics concepts was paired with teaching the students how to solve word problems (Fuchs et al. 2003).

Despite conflicting findings, results from several studies involving stimulant (mainly methylphenidate) and non-stimulant medication (mainly atomoxetine) treatment options for children with ADHD and SLD suggest both forms of medication may contribute to improved SLD outcomes. Although these medications do not directly target enhancement of reading, writing or mathematics skills, they play a role in supporting executive function (EF) skills, such as working memory, processing speed, and attentional focus (Grizenko et al. 2006; Bental and Tirosh 2008; Keulers et al. 2007; Tamm et al. 2017).

8.3.5 Example of Worksheets That Are Used in Schools to Check and Document That Appropriate Instruction in Reading Are Provided

8.3.5.1 Reading Worksheet

Suitable for all elementary, middle, and high school students who have been referred to special education due to a suspected learning disability that affects reading. Check if these areas are met:

Core General Education Language Arts Instruction

- Student has participated in daily general education reading/language arts instruction using the five areas of reading (e.g., through read-aloud; systematic phonics instruction; word study and structural analysis; fluency-building activities; explicit vocabulary instruction; literature think-aloud; comprehension strategy instruction. Small Group/Differentiated Instruction
- Student has participated in small group, differentiated reading instruction by the classroom teacher. Materials at the student's instructional level (90–95% word accuracy and at least 75–80% comprehension) have been used for a minimum of 4 days per week
- Progress Monitoring Assessments for the five areas of reading: phonemic awareness, phonics, fluency, vocabulary, and/or comprehension.
- Interventions have been implemented based on specific student needs in one or more of the five areas of reading: phonemic awareness, phonics, fluency, vocabulary, and/or comprehension.

If Decoding skills have been identified as an area of weakness:

- Student's phonemic awareness has been evaluated and if warranted, targeted interventions have been provided.
- Student has been provided with systematic, explicit phonics instruction.
- Student has been provided with regular opportunities to practice learned decoding skills in texts.

If a student's oral reading fluency has been identified as an area of weakness:

- Student's phonics skills have been evaluated and if warranted, targeted interventions have been provided.
- Student has been provided with regular opportunities to practice reading a variety of text at his/her independent level (at least 96% word accuracy and 90% comprehension).
- Student has been provided with teacher-directed fluency interventions focused specifically on improving oral reading fluency with connected text.
- If a student's reading comprehension skills have been identified as an area of weakness beyond what can be accounted for by identified decoding and/or reading fluency deficits:
- Student's vocabulary skills have been evaluated and if warranted, targeted interventions have been provided, with application to reading comprehension.
- Student's broad oral language skills (e.g., listening comprehension) have been evaluated and if warranted, targeted interventions have been provided, with application to reading comprehension.
- Student has been provided with explicit comprehension interventions (e.g., additional instruction in research based comprehension strategies such as summarization and use of graphic organizers; additional building of background knowledge and/or knowledge of text structure) to address his/her specific comprehension needs.

8.3.6 Example of Worksheets That Are Used in Schools to Check and Document That Appropriate Instruction in Mathematics Are Provided

8.3.6.1 Mathematics Worksheet

Check the areas that apply:

- Student participated in daily general education mathematics that involve a comprehensive, district-wide math curriculum that addresses state standards and all important areas of math, (e.g., through the explicit teaching of strategies that promote conceptual understanding, problem-solving, calculation skills, and procedural accuracy and fluency)
- Student has participated in small group, differentiated math instruction by the classroom teacher. Materials at the student's instructional level have been used for a minimum of 4 days per week

- Continuous progress monitoring has been provided to establish a basis for instructional decisions and to document a student's response to instruction. The targeted area may include math concepts, problem solving, calculation skills or procedural accuracy and fluency.

If calculation skills have been identified as an area of weakness:

- Student's conceptual understanding of numbers has been evaluated and if warranted, targeted interventions have been provided (e.g., additional, more explicit instruction with use of visual representations such as pictures or manipulatives).
- Student's automatic recall of facts has been evaluated and if warranted, targeted interventions have been provided.
- Student has been provided with explicit teaching of algorithms for calculation linking procedures to a conceptual understanding (e.g., written procedures for 2-digit subtraction with regrouping, long division).
- Student has been provided with regular opportunities to practice learned calculation skills in appropriate contexts, including cumulative review of previously learned skills.

If problem-solving skills have been identified as an area of weakness beyond what can be accounted for by identified calculation deficits and/or poor reading:

- Student's math-related vocabulary and other oral language skills have been evaluated and if warranted, targeted interventions have been provided, with application to math problem solving.
- Student's specific problem-solving skills (e.g., ability to determine which operation to use to solve a problem, identifying relevant vs. irrelevant information) have been evaluated and if warranted, targeted interventions have been provided.
- Student has been provided with regular opportunities to practice learned problem-solving skills, including cumulative review of previously learned skills.

8.3.7 Example of Worksheets That Are Used in Schools to Check and Document That Appropriate Instruction in Written Expression Are Provided

8.3.7.1 Written Expression Worksheet

Check the boxes that apply?

☐ Student has participated in daily general education written expression instruction General education instruction should involve all important areas of writing (e.g., through explicit teaching of basic writing skills, planning and organizational strategies, and writing knowledge; use of a writing process, with strategies for editing and revision; opportunities for practice; appropriate use of technology in writing; reading-writing connections).

☐ Student has participated in small group, differentiated written expression instruction by the classroom teacher as part of Tier I general education instruction (i.e., for all students). Materials appropriate to the student's instructional level have been used for a minimum of 4 days per week.

☐ Continuous progress monitoring has been provided to establish a basis for instructional decisions and to document a student's response to instruction in any of the following skills: basic writing skills, planning, text generation/content development, revisions.

☐ Supplemental scientific research-based interventions have been implemented based on specific student needs in important areas of writing, such as basic writing skills, text generation, or revision/editing processes.

If basic writing skills have been identified as an area of weakness:

- Student's basic writing skills (e.g., handwriting/keyboarding, spelling, capitalization, punctuation, sentence structure) have been evaluated and targeted interventions have been provided in specific areas of need.
- Student has been provided with appropriate access to and teaching about the use of technology in writing to improve basic writing skills (e.g., use of spell-checkers).
- Student has been taught strategies for reviewing and editing written work to improve basic writing skills. Student has been provided with regular opportunities to practice basic writing skills

If text generation (i.e., content aspects of writing that involve translating ideas into language) has been identified as an area of weakness, beyond what can be accounted for by identified weaknesses in basic writing skills:

- Student's vocabulary and other oral language skills have been evaluated and if warranted, targeted interventions have been provided, with application to writing.
- Student's ability to plan and organize writing have been evaluated and if warranted, targeted interventions have been provided (e.g., additional, more explicit teaching of strategies for brainstorming or researching ideas).
- Student's knowledge about writing (e.g., writing for an intended audience, use of formal vs. informal language in writing, schemas for different writing tasks such as reports vs. narratives) has been evaluated and if warranted, targeted interventions have been provided.
- Student has been provided with appropriate access to and teaching about the use of technology in writing to improve text generation (e.g., use of online thesaurus to improve word choice/avoid repetition of the same word).
- Student has been taught strategies for reviewing and revising written work to improve content/text generation.
- Student has been provided with regular opportunities to practice text generation.
- Sources
  2010 Guidelines for Identifying CHILDREN with Learning Disabilities by CONNECTICUT STATE DEPARTMENT OF EDUCATION

8.3.8 List Some Helpful Websites That Could Be Used to Educate Parents on Specific Learning Disorders?

National Center for Learning Disabilities (NCLD): www.understood.org; Accommodations: What They Are and How They Work

ADA-Americans with Disabilities Act—Testing Accommodations https://www.ada.gov/regs2014/testing_accommodations.pdf

Accommodations, Modifications, and Alternate Assessments: How They Affect Instruction and Assessment.

http://www.greatschools.org/gk/?s=accommodations

High-Stakes Assessment (Teaching LD) http://www.dldcec.org/ld_resources/alerts/4.htm

Forum on Accommodations in the 21st century: Critical Considerations for Students with Disabilities. Joint Publication of National Center on Educational Outcomes. https://nceo.umn.edu/docs/OnlinePubs/AccommodationsForumReport2011.pdf

References

American Psychiatric Association Diagnostic and statistical manual of mental disorders. Fourth Text Revision ed. Washington, DC: American Psychiatric Association; 2000.

Arnett AB, Pennington BF, Willcutt E, Dmitrieva J, Byrne B, Samuelsson S, et al. A cross-lagged model of the development of ADHD inattention symptoms and rapid naming speed. J Abnorm Child Psychol. 2012;40:1313–26.

Baker S, Gersten R, Lee D-S. A synthesis of empirical research on teaching mathematics to low-achieving students. Elem Sch J. 2002;103:51–73.

Bental B, Tirosh E. The effects of methylphenidate on word decoding accuracy in boys with attention-deficit/hyperactivity disorder. J Clin Psychopharmacol. 2008;28:89–92. https://doi.org/10.1097/jcp.0b013e3181603f0e.

Boada R, Willcutt EG, Pennington BF. Understanding the comorbidity between dyslexia and attention-deficit/hyperactivity disorder. Top Lang Disord. 2012;32:264–84.

Capano L, Minden D, Chen SX, Schacher RJ, Ickowicz A. Mathematical learning disorder in school-age children with attention-deficit hyperactivity disorder. Can J Psychiatr. 2008;53:392–9.

Compton DL, Fuchs D, Fuchs LS, Bryant JD. Selecting at-risk readers in first grade for early intervention: a two-year longitudinal study of decision rules and procedures. J Educ Psychol. 2006;98(2):394–409.

Duff FJ, Clarke PJ. Practitioner review: reading disorders: what are the effective interventions and how should they be implemented and evaluated? J Child Psychol Psychiatry. 2011;52(1):3–12. https://doi.org/10.1111/j.1469-7610.2010.02310.x. Epub 2010 Oct 7. Review. PubMed PMID: 21039483.

DuPaul G, Gormley MJ, Laracy SD. Comorbidity of LD and ADHD: implications of DSM-5 for assessment and treatment. J Learn Disabil. 2013;46:43–51.

Faraone SV, Perlis R, Doyle AE, et al. Molecular genetics of attention deficit hyperactivity disorder. Biol Psychiatr. 2005;57:1313–23.

Fletcher JM, Francis DJ, Morris RD, Lyon GR. Evidence-based assessment of learning disabilities in children and adolescents. J Clin Child Adolesc Psychol. 2005;34:506–22.

Fuchs D, Fuchs L. Peer-assisted learning strategies: promotion word recognition, fluency, and reading comprehension in young children. J Special Educ. 2005;39:34–44.

Fuchs LS, Fuchs D, Prentice K, et al. Explicitly teaching for transfer: effect on third-grade students' mathematical problem solving. J Educ Psychol. 2003;95:293–305.

Grizenko N, Bhat M, Schwartz G, Ter-Stepanian M, Joober R. Efficacy of methylphenidate in children with attention-deficit hyperactivity disorder and learning disabilities: a randomized crossover trial. J Psychiatry Neurosci. 2006;31:46–51.

Keulers EH, Hendriksen JG, Feron FJ, Wassenberg R, Wuisman-Frerker MG, Jolles J, et al. Methylphenidate improves reading performance in children with attention deficit hyperactivity disorder and comorbid dyslexia: an unblinded clinical trial. Eur J Paediatr Neurol. 2007;11:21–8. https://doi.org/10.1016/j.ejpn.2006.10.002.

Kim H, Schmidt KM, Murrah WM, Cameron CE, Grissmer D. A rasch analysis of the KeyMath-3 diagnostic assessment. J Appl Meas. 2015;16(4):365–78.

Melzer L, Pollica LS, Barzilla M. Executive function in the classroom: embedding strategy instruction into daily teaching practices. In: Meltzer L, editor. Executive function in education. New York: Guilford; 2007. p. 165–93.

Olson RK, Wise BW. Computer-based remediation for reading and related phonological disabilities. In: McKenna M, Labbo L, Kieffer R, Reinking D, editors. Handbook of literacy and technology, volume 2. Mahwah: Erlbaum; 2006. p. 57–74.

Pennington BF. From single to multiple deficit models of developmental disorders. Cognition. 2006;101:385–413.

Pham AV, Hasson RM. Verbal and visuospatial working memory as predictors of children's reading ability. Arch Clin Neuropsychol. 2014;29:467–77.

Pham AV, Riviere A. Specific learning disorders and ADHD: current issues in diagnosis across clinical and educational settings. Curr Psychiatry Rep. 2015;17(6):38.

Pitcher TM, Piek JP, Hay DA. Fine and gross motor ability in males with ADHD. Dev Med Child Neurol. 2003;45:525–35.

Rapin I. Dyscalculia and the calculating brain. Pediatr Neurol. 2016;61:11–20.

Re AM, Pedron M, Cornoldi C. Expressive writing difficulties in children described as exhibiting ADHD symptoms. J Learn Disabil. 2007;40:244–55.

Rosenberg J, Pennington BF, Willcutt EG, Olson RK. Gene by environment interactions influencing reading disability and the inattentive symptom dimension of attention deficit/hyperactivity disorder. J Child Psychol Psychiatry. 2012;53:243–51.

Semrud-Clikeman M, Bledsoe J. Updates on attention-deficit/hyperactivity disorder and learning disorders. Curr Psychiatry Rep. 2011;13(5):364–73.

Steele E, Lewandowski L, Rusling E. The effectiveness of bimodal text presentation for poor readers. Atlanta: National Association of School Psychologists; 1996.

Tamm L, Denton CA, Epstein JN, et al. Comparing treatments for children with ADHD and word reading difficulties: a randomized clinical trial. J Consult Clin Psychol. 2017;85(5):434–46.

Vellutino FR, Scanlon DM, Small S, Fanuele DP. Response to intervention as a vehicle for distinguishing between children with and without reading disabilities: evidence for the role of kindergarten and first-grade interventions. J Learn Disabil. 2006;39(2):157–69.

Yoshimasu K, Barbaresi WJ, Colligan RC, Killian JM, Voigt RG, Weaver AL, et al. Written-language disorder among children with and without ADHD in a population-based birth cohort. Pediatrics. 2011;128:e605–12.

ADHD and Depression 9

9.1 Objectives

- Describe the prevalence and morbidity of ADHD and Major Depressive disorders
- List some of the findings of the epidemiological data on ADHD and Suicide
- Discuss the relationship between ADHD and suicide
- Describe the possible explanations of the increased suicide risk in patients with ADHD
- Describe some of the challenges in diagnosis of ADHD in presence of depression or vice versa
- Discuss some of the management approaches of ADHD and Depression
- Understand the relationship between ADHD medication and Suicide
- Describe management approach to Suicidal Thoughts/Behaviour development during treatment with ADHD medications

9.2 What Are the Prevalence and Morbidity of ADHD and Depression?

Depression occurs in Youths with ADHD at a significantly higher rate than in Youths without ADHD. Youths with ADHD and depression together have a more severe course of psychopathology and a higher risk of long-term impairment and suicide than youths with either disorder alone (Daviss 2008).

The prevalence rate of ADHD in patients with major depressive disorder ranges from 5 to 16% in several studies (Bond et al. 2012).

A study concluded that a total of 10–40% of children and adolescents with ADHD show comorbid affective disorders, mostly depression with the symptomatology of low or irritated mood, loss of interest and pleasure in usually enjoyable activities, sleep disturbances, reduced appetite etc. (Milberger et al. 1995).

Depressive disorders in youths with ADHD may typically occur several years after the onset of ADHD (Biederman et al. 1995).

J. Sadek, *Clinician's Guide to ADHD Comorbidities in Children and Adolescents*,
https://doi.org/10.1007/978-3-319-45635-5_9

Common notion is that the cumulative effects of ADHD-related impairments and the negative environmental circumstances triggered by these may lead some youths with ADHD to eventually develop depression (Goodman and Thase 2009).

ADHD and depression are highly impairing disorders, however the comorbidity of both conditions results in even greater levels of psychosocial impairment (Biederman et al. 2008).

Presence of ADHD in a prospective study of females ± ADHD aged 6–18 years, after a follow-up period of 5 years, detected an earlier age of onset of depression, a longer duration of depressive episodes and higher rates of suicidality and hospitalization compared to patients with "depression only" (Biederman et al. 2008).

Persistence of major depression could not be predicted by severity of ADHD (Daviss et al. 2008).

9.3 What Are Some of the Findings of the Epidemiological Data on ADHD and Suicide?

In the United Kingdom the rate of self-harm in 11–15-year olds with hyperkinetic disorder was 8.5%, (Furczyk and Thome 2014).

ADHD was found to occur more frequently in suicidal groups than control group (Impey and Heun 2012).

A large population based study in Sweden found that individuals with ADHD had an increased risk of both attempted and completed suicide compared with matched control participants (OR = 8.46 [95% CI, 8.07–8.87] and OR = 12.22 [95% CI, 8.67–17.22], respectively), even after adjusting for comorbid psychiatric disorders (OR = 3.62 [95% CI, 3.29–3.98] and OR = 5.91 [95% CI, 2.45–14.27], respectively (Ljung et al. 2014 JAMA).

9.4 What Is the Relationship Between ADHD and Suicide?

ADHD is associated with an increased risk of both attempted and completed suicide.

While ADHD can be viewed as an independent risk factor for suicide, some authors suggest that the association ADHD and suicide is mediated by the symptoms of comorbid disorders as mood or anxiety disorders (Balazs et al. 2014).

Recent study suggested that ADHD symptoms were linked to suicidal behavior after controlling for comorbid conditions (Stickley et al. 2016).

9.5 What Are the Possible Explanations of the Increased Suicide Risk in Patients with ADHD?

9.5.1 Comorbid Disorders

Some authors reported significant associations between ADHD and several psychiatric disorders.

ADHD patients compared to controls are more likely to have psychiatric comorbidity and more likely to attempt suicide. Examples of comorbid disorders with ADHD:

Alcohol, substance and nicotine use disorders.
Mood disorders, major depressive disorder, bipolar disorder.
Anxiety disorders, obsessive–compulsive disorder, post-traumatic stress disorder and phobia.
Somatoform disorder and sleep disorders (Park et al. 2011; Keresztény et al. 2012; Murphy et al. 2002).

Comorbid depression and ADHD predisposed to more lethal suicide attempts and greater desire to end their life (Nasser and Overholser 1999) and associated with a higher rate of suicidal ideation and attempts (Biederman et al. 2008; Patros et al. 2013).

Substance abuse, co-occurring with ADHD, is associated with an increased risk of suicide and suicide attempts (Arias et al. 2008; Huntley et al. 2012).

9.5.2 Cognitive Impairment and Personality Traits

Impaired decision-making is a vulnerability for suicidal behavior (Jollant et al. 2007) and ADHD (Masunami et al. 2009; Miller et al. 2013).

Poor decision making can be a result of the impulsivity which is an important symptom of ADHD.

One study suggested that the personality trait of impulsivity contributed to attempting suicide (Swann et al. 2008).

9.5.3 Neurobiology

Lower cerebrospinal fluid concentration of the dopamine metabolite homovanillic acid (HVA), as well as of the serotonin metabolite 5-hydroxyindoleacetic acid (5-HIAA) (Asberg et al. 1976) have been suggested to be a possible underlying mechanism in suicide and ADHD.

A decreased level of dopamine in one of the components of the reward system, specifically the nucleus accumbens, was found to be low in the post-mortem brains of depressed suicide patients and also in ADHD patients (Bowden et al. 1997).

A recent large population based study in Sweden suggested that there is an increased risk of both attempted and completed suicide in ADHD patients and their first degree relatives. The study suggested that shared genetic factors are important for this association and that individuals with ADHD and their family members are important targets for suicide prevention and treatment. Ongoing research is needed in that area.

9.6 What Are Some of the Challenges in Diagnosis of ADHD in Presence of Depression or Vice Versa?

Symptom overlap between ADHD and MDD may lead to misdiagnosis. Some of the DSM-V criteria for diagnosis of MDD might be associated with ADHD to some degree such as poor concentration, insomnia, psychomotor agitation or retardation and fatigue. On the other hand Inattentive symptoms of ADHD such as distractibility, difficulty sustaining attention or hyperactivity symptoms such as difficulty sitting still might mimic symptoms of depression. It is important to make the distinction between demoralization, an outgrowth of the negative consequences of ADHD, and a clinical diagnosis of major depression that is episodic (Goodman et al. 2008).

9.7 What Are the Management Approaches of ADHD and Depression?

Some evidence suggests that ADHD treatments may be less effective in patients with active depression and may lead to an exacerbation of dysphoria, poor sleep, and decreased appetite (Weiss and Hechtman 2006).

In patients with moderate to severe Depression and ADHD, some clinical guidelines recommend to start by assessing for suicide risk and treating depression first (CADDRA 2018).

In patients with mild depression and ADHD, the recommendations suggest to continue to assess for suicide risk, start ADHD treatment and add an antidepressant when indicated (CADDRA 2018). Stimulants appeared to be effective for the treatment of ADHD symptoms in children with mild to moderate depressive symptoms (Kunwar et al. 2007).

There is increasing evidence for the efficacy of selective serotoninergic reuptake inhibitors (SSRIs) in treating pediatric major depressive disorder (MDD) in general (Birmaher et al. 2007) but had limited benefit for ADHD symptoms (Daviss 2008). Some researchers reported risk factors for developing bipolar disorder among depressed youth that included rapid onset, psychomotor retardation, psychotic features, a family history of unipolar depression or bipolar disorder and a history of antidepressant induced mania (AIM) (Goldberg and Truman 2003).

Atomoxetine which is a Noradrenergic reuptake inhibitor (NRI) demonstrates an efficacy for ADHD symptoms with a moderate effect size of 0.63 but limited results for treatment of depression (Bangs et al. 2007).

Since SSRIs are metabolized in the liver, while 80% of methylphenidate is metabolized extrahepatically, there has been little concern with this combination (Greenhill et al. 2002).

Cognitive Behavioural Therapy may be helpful in patient with depression and ADHD and often in conjunction with medications. Other psychosocial treatments for ADHD can also be employed such as organizational skills, anger management training, social skills and education about the illness and the medication (CADDRA 2018).

9.8 What Is the Relationship Between ADHD Medication and Suicide?

9.8.1 Atomoxetine

In 2005, both the United States Food and Drug Administration and Health Canada warned of increased rates of suicidal ideation among patients taking atomoxetine in placebo-controlled trials. The later published meta-analysis that prompted the warnings after reviewing 12 studies comparing outcomes in children treated with atomoxetine or placebo. Suicidal ideation was reported to have occurred in 5 (0.37%) of 1357 children given atomoxetine, but in none of 851 children receiving placebo (Bangs et al. 2008).

As a result, health providers were advised to closely monitor children and adolescents treated with atomoxetine for aggravation of symptoms such as agitation, irritability, suicidal thinking or behaviours and unusual changes in behaviour.

A case report was published in 2008 of acute agitation and suicidal ideation in an 11-year-old boy after commencing atomoxetine (Paxton and Cranswick 2008).

9.8.2 Stimulant Medications

One study that examined the adult outcomes of childhood stimulant medication in a relatively small group of 32 subjects, found that for 20 young adults, the childhood treatment had no lasting effect, but for 11 others, the positive effects lasted long after treatment was discontinued. Higher dosage of medication was associated with fewer diagnoses of alcoholism and with fewer suicide attempts (Paternite et al. 1999).

There are seven comparator trials of atomoxetine and methylphenidate, five of which were randomised double blind and included in the analysis of suicide risk while receiving ADHD medications. In total there were five events using FDA coding 1–4, atomoxetine 3/559; Methylphenidate 2/465. All events using FDA coding 1–4 were suicidal ideation: there were no suicide attempts nor completed suicides and there was no difference in risk between atomexetine and methylphenidate with a Mantel-Haenszel risk ratio of 0.52 (95% CI; 0.06, 4.54). Mantel-Haenszel risk ratio (MH) used for categorical data replacing the odds ratio(OR) (Bushe and Savill 2013).

9.9 What Do I Tell Patients and Families When Asked About Suicide and ADHD Medication?

Some patients may inquire about suicide risk when taking ADHD medications particularly in North America after Health Canada Announcement in March 2015: "ADHD drugs may increase risk of suicidal thoughts and behaviours in some people; benefits still outweigh risks".

Health Canada reported increased risk of suicidal ideation when the ADHD medication was started, when the dose was changed and when the medication was stopped. Mood symptoms may be induced by psychostimulants (irritability, dysphoria).

It was suggested that while patients and their families should be made aware of the increased risk of suicidal thoughts and behaviours among people who have ADHD, families should also be told this strong warning on ADHD medications should not be a cause for panic and that:

- Patients taking ADHD medications, as well as their parents, families and friends, should monitor for suicidal thoughts and behaviours.
- Patients and families be encouraged to report any distressing thoughts or feelings immediately to their doctor. This applies at all stages of treatment and even after ADHD therapy has been stopped.
- ADHD medication should not be changed or stopped without medical advice
- Healthcare professionals monitor patients more closely around the start of treatment, at dose change and when medication is stopped.
- Suicide risk assessment for patients at moderate or high risk of suicide is essential and a clear management plan should be developed (CADDRA 2018).

9.10 Give Examples of Questions That Can Be Asked to Screen for Suicide?

Example #1 Intro: "I'm going to ask you a few quick questions about how you think and feel right now."

"Sometimes when people are very upset, they think about hurting themselves. Has this happened to you? Do you feel that way now? Was there ever another time you felt that way?

Example #2 Sometimes people who get upset or feel bad, wish they were dead or feel they'd be better off dead. Have you ever felt like life is not worth living? Do you feel that way now? Did these thoughts start after you took the medication?

9.11 How Should I Manage Suicidal Thoughts/Behaviour During Treatment with ADHD Medications?

- Psychiatric history should be taken; this should routinely include an assessment of suicidality, either via general enquiry or via a standardized suicidality rating tool.
- Observe patients for the emergence of depression, irritability and suicidal ideation as part of the routine monitoring. Determine whether the patient is expressing suicidal ideation, intent, plan or is there a history of chronic self-harm behavior as in a personality disorder.

- Families and caregivers should be advised of the need to recognize any appearance of emotional change, self-injurious thinking, suicidal ideation and irritability.
- Caution is required when prescribing ADHD drugs to patients with a past history of serious suicidal attempt or current untreated severe and impairing depression.
- In the case of ADHD and concurrent suicidal ideation in the context of a major depressive episode, the clinician should focus initially on the treatment of the disorder that is the most severe and impairing, i.e. the depressive disorder and its potentially life threatening complications (e.g., suicidality).
- If suicidal ideation emerges during ADHD treatment, urgent psychiatric evaluation should be arranged.
- Consideration should be given to reducing the dose and/or other changes in the therapeutic regimen, including the possibility of discontinuing the medication, especially if these symptoms are severe or abrupt in onset, or were not part of the patient's presenting symptoms.
- It should, however, not automatically be assumed that any suicidal ideation or attempt is an adverse effect of medication.

References on Depression and Suicide

Arias AJ, et al. Correlates of co-occurring ADHD in drug dependent subjects: prevalence and features of substance dependence and psychiatric disorders. Addict Behav. 2008;33(9):1199–207.

Asberg M, Träskman L, Thorén P. 5-HIAA in the cerebrospinal fluid. A biochemical suicide predictor? Arch Gen Psychiatry. 1976;33(10):1193–7.

Balazs J, Miklósi M, Keresztény A, Dallos G, Gádoros J. Attention-deficit hyperactivity disorder and suicidality in a treatment naïve sample of children and adolescents. J Affect Disord. 2014;152–154:282–7.

Bangs ME, Emslie GJ, Spencer TJ, et al. Atomoxetine ADHD and Comorbid MDD Study Group. Efficacy and safety of atomoxetine in adolescents with attention-deficit/hyperactivity disorder and major depression. J Child Adolesc Psychopharmacol. 2007;17(4):407–20.

Bangs ME, et al. Meta-analysis of suicide-related behavior events in patients treated with atomoxetine. J Am Acad Child Adolesc Psychiatry. 2008;47(2):209–18.

Biederman J, Faraone S, Mick E, Lelon E. Psychiatric comorbidity among referred juveniles with major depression: fact or artifact? J Am Acad Child Adolesc Psychiatry. 1995;34:579–90.

Biederman J, et al. New insights into the comorbidity between ADHD and major depression in adolescent and young adult females. J Am Acad Child Adolesc Psychiatry. 2008;47(4):426–34.

Birmaher B, Brent D, AACAP Work Group on Quality Issues, Bernet W, Bukstein O, Walter H, Benson RS, Chrisman A, Farchione T, Greenhill L, Hamilton J, Keable H, Kinlan J, Schoettle U, Stock S, Ptakowski KK, Medicus J. Practice parameter for the assessment and treatment of children and adolescents with depressive disorders. J Am Acad Child Adolesc Psychiatry. 2007;46(11):1503–26.

Bond DJ, Hadjipavlou G, Lam RW, et al. Canadian Network for Mood and Anxiety Treatments (CANMAT) Task Force. The Canadian Network for Mood and Anxiety Treatments (CANMAT) task force recommendations for the management of patients with mood disorders and comorbid attention-deficit/hyperactivity disorder. Ann Clin Psychiatry. 2012;24(1):23–37.

Bowden C, Cheetham SC, Lowther S, Katona CL, Crompton MR, Horton RW. Reduced dopamine turnover in the basal ganglia of depressed suicides. Brain Res. 1997;769(1):135–40.

Bushe CJ, Savill NC. Suicide related events and attention deficit hyperactivity disorder treatments in children and adolescents: a meta-analysis of atomoxetine and methylphenidate comparator clinical trials. Child Adolesc Psychiatry Ment Health. 2013;7:19.

CADDRA. Canadian ADHD practice guidelines. 4th ed. 2018. https://www.caddra.ca/wp-content/uploads/CADDRA-Guidelines-4th-Edition_-Feb2018.pd

Daviss WB. A review of co-morbid depression in pediatric ADHD: etiology, phenomenology, and treatment. J Child Adolesc Psychopharmacol. 2008;18(6):565–71.

Daviss WB, Birmaher B, Diler RS, Mintz J. Does pharmacotherapy for attention-deficit/hyperactivity disorder predict risk of later major depression? J Child Adolesc Psychopharmacol. 2008;18:257–64.

Furczyk K, Thome J. Adult ADHD and suicide. Atten Defic Hyperact Disord. 2014;6(3):153–8.

Goldberg JF, Truman CJ. Antidepressant-induced mania: an overview of current controversies. Bipolar Disord. 2003;5(6):407–20.

Goodman DW, Thase ME. Recognizing ADHD in adults with comorbid mood disorders: implications for identification and management. Postgrad Med. 2009;121(5):20–30.

Goodman G, Gerstadt C, Pfeffer CR, Stroh M, Valdez A. ADHD and aggression as correlates of suicidal behavior in assaultive prepubertal psychiatric inpatients. Suicide Life Threat Behav. 2008;38(1):46–59.

Greenhill LL, Pliszka S, Dulcan MK, et al. American Academy of Child and Adolescent Psychiatry. Practice parameter for the use of stimulant medications in the treatment of children, adolescents, and adults. J Am Acad Child Adolesc Psychiatry. 2002;41(2 Suppl):26S–49S.

Huntley Z, et al. Rates of undiagnosed attention deficit hyperactivity disorder in London drug and alcohol detoxification units. BMC Psychiatry. 2012;6(12):223.

Impey M, Heun R. Completed suicide, ideation and attempt in attention deficit hyperactivity disorder. Acta Psychiatr Scand. 2012;125(2):93–102.

Jollant F, Guillaume S, Jaussent I, Castelnau D, Malafosse A, Courtet P. Impaired decision-making in suicide attempters may increase the risk of problems in affective relationships. J Affect Disord. 2007;99(1–3):59–62. Epub 2006 Sep 28. PubMed PMID: 17010445.

Keresztény A, Dallos G, Miklósi M, Róka A, Gádoros J, Balázs J. Comparing the comorbidity of attention-deficit/hyperactivity disorder in childhood and adolescence. Psychiatr Hung. 2012;27(3):165–73.

Kunwar A, Dewan M, Faraone SV. Treating common psychiatric disorders associated with attention-deficit/hyperactivity disorder. Expert Opin Pharmacother. 2007;8:555–6.

Ljung T, Chen Q, Lichtenstein P, Larsson H. Common etiological factors of attention-deficit/hyperactivity disorder and suicidal behavior: a population-based study in Sweden. JAMA Psychiat. 2014;71(8):958–64.

Masunami T, Okazaki S, Maekawa H. Decision-making patterns and sensitivity to reward and punishment in children with attention-deficit hyperactivity disorder. Int J Psychophysiol. 2009;72(3):283–8.

Milberger S, Biederman J, Faraone SV, Murphy J, Tsuang MT. Attention deficit hyperactivity disorder and comorbid disorders: issues of overlapping symptoms. Am J Psychiatry. 1995;152:1793–9.

Miller M, Sheridan M, Cardoos SL, Hinshaw SP. Impaired decision-making as a young adult outcome of girls diagnosed with attention-deficit/hyperactivity disorder in childhood. J Int Neuropsychol Soc. 2013;19(1):110–4.

Murphy KR, Barkley RA, Bush T. Young adults with attention deficit hyperactivity disorder: subtype differences in comorbidity, educational, and clinical history. J Nerv Ment Dis. 2002;190(3):147–57.

Nasser EH, Overholser JC. Assessing varying degrees of lethality in depressed adolescent suicide attempters. Acta Psychiatr Scand. 1999;99(6):423–31.

Park S, et al. Prevalence, correlates, and comorbidities of adult ADHD symptoms in Korea: results of the Korean epidemiologic catchment area study. Psychiatry Res. 2011;186(2–3):378–83.

Paternite CE, Loney J, Salisbury H, Whaley MA. Childhood inattention-overactivity, aggression, and stimulant medication history as predictors of young adult outcomes. J Child Adolesc Psychopharmacol. 1999;9(3):169–84.

Patros CH, Hudec KL, Alderson RM, Kasper LJ, Davidson C, Wingate LR. Symptoms of attention-deficit/hyperactivity disorder (ADHD) moderate suicidal behaviors in college students with depressed mood. J Clin Psychol. 2013;69(9):980–93.

Paxton GA, Cranswick NE. Acute suicidality after commencing atomoxetine. J Paediatr Child Health. 2008;44(10):596–8.

Stickley A, Koyanagi A, Ruchkin V, Kamio Y. Attention-deficit/hyperactivity disorder symptoms and suicide ideation and attempts: findings from the Adult Psychiatric Morbidity Survey 2007. J Affect Disord. 2016;189:321–8.

Swann AC, Steinberg JL, Lijffijt M, Moeller FG. Impulsivity: differential relationship to depression and mania in bipolar disorder. J Affect Disord. 2008;106(3):241–8. Epub 2007 Sep 5. PubMed PMID: 17822778.

Weiss M, Hechtman L. Adult ADHD Research Group. A randomized double-blind trial of paroxetine and/or dextroamphetamine and problem-focused therapy for attention-deficit/hyperactivity disorder in adults. J Clin Psychiatry. 2006;67(4):611–9.

ADHD and Bipolar Disorder

10

10.1 Objectives

- Discuss the prevalence rate of ADHD versus Bipolar Disorder in late adolescence
- List some of the challenges in differentiating Bipolar disorder from ADHD in late adolescence
- Describe the explanatory theories regarding comorbid bipolar disorder and ADHD
- Describe some of the clinical features that help in clarifying the diagnosis of ADHD and BD in late adolescence
- Describe the management approaches to comorbid bipolar disorder and ADHD in in late adolescence

10.2 Questions

10.2.1 What Is the Prevalence Rate of ADHD Versus Bipolar Disorder in Late Adolescence?

The prevalence of ADHD in youths (1.9%) is considerably higher than that of episodic DSM-IV bipolar disorder (0.1%) (Leibenluft 2011).

J. Sadek, *Clinician's Guide to ADHD Comorbidities in Children and Adolescents*,
https://doi.org/10.1007/978-3-319-45635-5_10

10.2.2 What Are Some of the Challenges in Differentiating Bipolar Disorder from ADHD?

Some challenges are related to the following issues (Leibenluft 2011; Marangoni et al. 2015):

- Both disorders have a young age of onset (ADHD may manifest earlier)
- Youths with severe irritability but without distinct manic episodes could be misdiagnosed with bipolar disorder despite having symptoms of disruptive mood dysregulation disorder (Leibenluft 2011)
- Youths with severe mood dysregulation, compared to those with bipolar disorder and/or healthy comparison subjects, may have reduced attentional interference from emotional distracters (Leibenluft 2011).
- Some patients have limited ability to self-report symptoms
- ADHD and mania diagnostically share nonspecific symptoms (distractibility, motoric hyperactivity, and talkativeness
- ADHD and Bipolar disorder share several similar psychiatric comorbidities such as anxiety, disruptive behavior disorders, and substance use disorder.
- Euthymic youths with bipolar disorder exhibit significant cognitive dysfunction encompassing verbal learning and memory, working memory, and/or visual learning and memory domains (Elias et al. 2017).
- The course of bipolar disorder in youth may have less clear episodic course than adults.

10.2.3 List Some of the Medical Conditions That Imitate Bipolar Disorder?

Medical conditions imitating bipolar disorder may include migraine, multiple sclerosis, neoplasm, epilepsy especially temporal lobe, cerebrovascular disorders, head trauma, thyroid dysfunction, pheochromocytoma, AIDS, brain abscess, bacterial and viral infections, Hepatic encephalopathy, Wilson disease, chronic lung disease, systemic lupus erythematosus, chronic lung disease, alcohol or substance intoxication or withdrawal and medications.

10.2.4 What Are the Clinical Features That May Help in Clarifying the Diagnosis of ADHD and Bipolar Disorder?

In most uncomplicated cases in late adolescence, the discrete appearance of high mood, decrease need for sleep, and grandiosity are more likely to predict a diagnosis of BD, especially if impulsive behavior is exhibited around money (spending); sex (promiscuity); and substances (tobacco, alcohol, substances).

On the other hand, fidgeting and restlessness and inefficient and disorganized performances stemming from inattentiveness, distractibility and forgetfulness, often point to ADHD (Jensen et al. 2001).

The following table may help clarify the diagnosis (Marangoni et al. 2015):

Symptoms	ADHD	Bipolar disorder in youth >16
Suicide	Not a diagnostic feature	Suicidal thoughts, plans and attempts are common
Mood	Stable mood or presence of mood symptoms secondary to academic or social difficulties or demoralization.	In mania: high or irritable mood In depression: Low or irritable mood associated with poor or increased appetite
Hyperactivity	High, but relatively stable levels of locomotor activity Restlessness, fidgeting, and hyperactive behavior	Periods of intense hyperactivity or agitation in mania. Periods of low activity, exhaustion and boredom during depressive episodes
Grandiosity	Usually Not present	Present in manic episodes
Energy	Less fluctuation in energy level	circadian rhythms are altered, resulting in greater fluctuations of energy and activity
Speech	Talkative due to lack of inhibition, may be sometimes redirected	Pressure of speech due to flight of ideas and vivid imagination
Sleep	No decreased need for sleep Early insomnia commonly present Middle and late insomnia, commonly NOT observed	Decreased need for sleep Early insomnia commonly present Middle and late insomnia, commonly observed
Psychosis	Do not exhibit psychotic symptoms	Can present with psychotic symptoms
Effect of lithium/ mood stabilizers	Lithium/mood stabilizers have no effect	Lithium/mood stabilizers help symptoms
Effect of stimulants	Stimulants are effective	Stimulants can disrupt sleep/mood
Impulsivity	Hypersexual behavior is not part of the ADHD clinical presentation.	Sexual behaviors (both self-stimulation and towards others) has been described in some adolescents with BD. Common impulsive substance use
Dysphoria, crying spells, temper tantrums, and mood lability	Not described as precursor of ADHD	Can be part of disruptive mood dysregulation disorder
Cycling	Not common	Commonly described in youth bipolar disorder
Academic performance	Difficulties with inattention, failure to complete homework, and poor concentration often interfere with academic achievement consistently over time and across subjects.	More variable, uneven academic performance performances coinciding with periods of emotional instability and especially depressive phases or periods of increased anxiety and school refusal

Symptoms	ADHD	Bipolar disorder in youth >16
Somatic Complaints	Not common	Common particularly with depression
Aggressive behavior	Less common except if comorbid with conduct disorder	More common
Family history	Adoption and twin studies estimate that 60–80% of the risk for ADHD is heritable,	Most significant risk factor for developing BD is a positive family history. Heritability 58–85%

10.2.5 What Are the Management Approaches to Comorbid Bipolar Disorder and ADHD in Late Adolescence?

The treatment plan for youth above age 16 should include pharmacological and psychosocial treatment for each disorder and bipolar disorder should be treated first (Perugi et al. 2017).

National Institute for Health and Care Excellence (NICE) in UK recommends that when offering treatment to older adolescents with bipolar disorder, take into account their cognitive ability, emotional maturity, developmental level, their capacity to consent to treatment, the severity of their bipolar disorder and risk of suicide or self-harm or any other risk. They also recommend that during the treatment of manic episode, do not offer Valproate to girls or young women of childbearing potential (NICE 2015).

10.2.5.1 Pharmacological Treatment

Combination treatment is often required for treatment of comorbidity of bipolar disorder and ADHD.

Mood-stabilizing agents and atypical antipsychotic may be beneficial for bipolar disorder in late adolescence but are unlikely to enhance attention in patients with ADHD and should be monitored due to their associated with serious side effects (Dols et al. 2013; Young et al. 2015).

Presence of ADHD comorbidity in patients with bipolar disorder may be a predictor of poorer treatment response (Masi et al. 2012).

Some researchers recommended not to prescribe stimulants in patients with bipolar disorder in absence of mood stabilizers and if stimulants are used patients should be regularly assessed for possible manic, or mixed symptoms. The addition of a psychostimulant or atomoxetine to treat co-morbid ADHD appears generally beneficial. However, adolescents with bipolar disorder and ADHD may still react to psychostimulants or atomoxetine with development or exacerbation of manic symptoms (Goldsmith et al. 2011; Perugi et al. 2017). Researchers suggested that regular monitoring is required and if manic episode develops, stimulants should be stopped ((Goldsmith et al. 2011).

Stimulants have been shown to be ineffective in the treatment of bipolar disorder, can cause disruption of sleep and circadian rhythms, and may also cause psychotic symptoms (Berman et al. 2009; Clavenna and Bonati 2014; Goldsmith et al. 2011).

In general, the recommendations on pharmacological treatment of comorbid ADHD and Bipolar disorder remains controversial due to the limited number of studies in this area.

10.2.5.2 Psychosocial Treatment

Psychosocial treatment for older adolescents with bipolar disorder may include multi-family psychoeducation groups; family-focused treatment (FFT), multifamily and individual family psychoeducational psychotherapy (MF-PEP and IF-PEP), dialectical behavior therapy, and interpersonal and social rhythm therapy (West and Pavuluri 2009; Fristad et al. 2009; Fristad and MacPherson 2014).

Psychosocial treatments for ADHD in adolescence include psychoeducation, cognitive behavioral therapy, behavior contingency management, motivational enhancement, and academic, organizational, and social skills training techniques (Chan et al. 2016).

A review by Mongia M, Hechtman L concluded that CBT is a feasible and acceptable treatment strategy in medicated adults with ADHD that leads to improvement in ADHD symptoms and co-morbid problems (Mongia and Hechtman 2012).

References

Bipolar Disorders

Berman SM, Kuczenski R, McCracken JT, London ED. Potential adverse effects of amphetamine treatment on brain and behavior: a review. Mol Psychiatry. 2009;14(2):123–42.

Chan E, Fogler JM, Hammerness PG. Treatment of attention-deficit/hyperactivity disorder in adolescents: a systematic review. JAMA. 2016;315(18):1997–2008.

Clavenna A, Bonati M. Safety of medicines used for ADHD in children: a review of published prospective clinical trials. Arch Dis Child. 2014;99(9):866–72.

Dols A, Sienaert P, van Gerven H, Schouws S, Stevens A, Kupka R, et al. The prevalence and management of side effects of lithium and anticonvulsants as mood stabilizers in bipolar disorder from a clinical perspective: a review. Int Clin Psychopharmacol. 2013;28(6):287–96.

Elias LR, Miskowiak KW, Vale AM, Köhler CA, Kjærstad HL, Stubbs B, Kessing LV, Vieta E, Maes M, Goldstein BI, Carvalho AF. Cognitive impairment in euthymic pediatric bipolar disorder: a systematic review and meta-analysis. J Am Acad Child Adolesc Psychiatry. 2017;56(4):286–96.

Fristad MA, MacPherson HA. Evidence-based psychosocial treatments for child and adolescent bipolar spectrum disorders. J Clin Child Adolesc Psychol. 2014;43(3):339–55.

Fristad MA, Verducci JS, Walters K, Young ME. Impact of multifamily psychoeducational psychotherapy in treating children aged 8 to 12 years with mood disorders. Arch Gen Psychiatry. 2009;66(9):1013–21.

Goldsmith M, Singh M, Chang K. Antidepressants and psychostimulants in pediatric populations: is there an association with mania? Paediatr Drugs. 2011;13(4):225–43.

Jensen P, Hinshaw SP, Swanson JM, Greenhill LL, Conners CK, Arnold LE, et al. Findings from the NIMH Multi-modal Treatment Study (MTA): implications and applications for primary care providers. J Dev Behav Pediatr. 2001;22(1):60–73.

Leibenluft E. Severe mood dysregulation, irritability, and the diagnostic boundaries of bipolar disorder in youths. Am J Psychiatry. 2011;168(2):129–42.

Marangoni C, De Chiara L, Faedda GL. Bipolar disorder and ADHD: comorbidity and diagnostic distinctions. Curr Psychiatry Rep. 2015;17(8):604.

Masi G, Mucci M, Pfanner C, Berloffa S, Magazù A, Perugi G. Developmental pathways for different subtypes of early-onset bipolarity in youths. J Clin Psychiatry. 2012;73(10):1335–41.

Mongia M, Hechtman L. Cognitive behavior therapy for adults with attention-deficit/hyperactivity disorder: a review of recent randomized controlled trials. Curr Psychiatry Rep. 2012;14(5):561–7.

National Institute for Health and Care Excellence (NICE) Guidelines 2015.

Perugi G, Vannucchi G, Bedani F, Favaretto E. Use of stimulants in bipolar disorder. Curr Psychiatry Rep. 2017;19(1):7.

West AE, Pavuluri MN. Psychosocial treatments for childhood and adolescent bipolar disorder. Child Adolesc Psychiatr Clin N Am. 2009;18(2):471–82, x–xi.

Young SL, Taylor M, Lawrie SM. 'First do no harm'. A systematic review of the prevalence and management of antipsychotic adverse effects. J Psychopharmacol. 2015;29(4):353–62.

Bibliography

Barbaresi WJ, et al. Mortality, ADHD, and psychosocial adversity in adults with childhood ADHD: a prospective study. Pediatrics. 2013;131(4):637–44.

Carlat DA. Evidence based somatic treatment of depression in adults. Psychiatr Clin North Am. 2012;35:131–42.

Chen Q, Sjölander A, Runeson B, D'Onofrio BM, Lichtenstein P, Larsson H. Drug treatment for attention-deficit/hyperactivity disorder and suicidal behaviour: register based study. BMJ. 2014;348:g3769.

Chronis-Tuscano A, et al. Very early predictors of adolescent depression and suicide attempts in children with attention deficit/hyperactivity disorder. Arch Gen Psychiatry. 2010;67(10):1044–51.

Corruble E, et al. Defense styles, impulsivity and suicide attempts in major depression. Psychopathology. 2003;36(6):279–84.

Daviss WB, Birmaher B, Diler RS, Mintz J. Does pharmacotherapy for attention-deficit/hyperactivity disorder predict risk of later major depression? J Child Adolesc Psychopharmacol. 2008;18:257–64.

Dougherty LR, Smith VC, Bufferd SJ, Carlson GA, Stringaris A, Leibenluft E, Klein DN. DSM-5 disruptive mood dysregulation disorder: correlates and predictors in young children. Psychol Med. 2014;44(11):2339–50.

Evans C, Blackburn D, Butt P, Dattani D. Use and abuse of methylphenidate in attention-deficit/hyperactivity disorder. Beware of legitimate prescriptions being diverted. Can Pharm J. 2004;137(6):30–5.

Eyre O, Langley K, Stringaris A, Leibenluft E, Collishaw S, Thapar A. Irritability in ADHD: associations with depression liability. J Affect Disord. 2017;215:281–7.

Findling RL. Open-label treatment of comorbid depression and attentional disorders with co-administration of serotonin reuptake inhibitors and psychostimulants in children, adolescents, and adults: a case series. J Child Adolesc Psychopharmacol. 1996 Fall;6(3):165–75.

Goldston DB, et al. Psychiatric diagnoses as contemporaneous risk factors for suicide attempts among adolescents and young adults: developmental changes. J Consult Clin Psychol. 2009;77(2):281–90.

Graham J, et al. European guidelines on managing adverse effects of medication for ADHD. Eur Child Adolesc Psychiatry. 2011;20(1):17–37.
Greening L, et al. Pathways to suicidal behaviors in childhood. Suicide Life Threat Behav. 2008;38(1):35–45.
Hardy SE. Methylphenidate for the treatment of depressive symptoms, including fatigue and apathy, in medically ill older adults and terminally ill adults. Am J Geriatr Pharmacother. 2009 Feb;7(1):34–59.
Hinshaw SP. Prospective follow-up of girls with attentiondeficit/hyperactivity disorder into early adulthood: continuing impairment includes elevated risk for suicide attempts and self injury. J Consult Clin Psychol. 2012;80(6):1041–51.
Kircanski K, Zhang S, Stringaris A, Wiggins JL, Towbin KE, Pine DS, Leibenluft E, Brotman MA. Empirically derived patterns of psychiatric symptoms in youth: a latent profile analysis. J Affect Disord. 2017;216:109–16.
Klein-Schwartz W. Abuse and toxicity of methylphenidate. Curr Opin Pediatr. 2002;14(2):219–23. Review. PubMed PMID: 11981294
McCarthy S, Cranswick N, Potts L, Taylor E, Wong IC. Mortality associated with attention-deficit hyperactivity disorder (ADHD) drug treatment: a retrospective cohort study of children, adolescents and young adults using the general practice research database. Drug Saf. 2009;32(11):1089–96.
Meinzer MC, Pettit JW, Viswesvaran C. The co-occurrence of attention-deficit/hyperactivity disorder and unipolar depression in children and adolescents: a meta-analytic review. Clin Psychol Rev. 2014;34(8):595–607.
Nicoli M, Bouchez S, Nieto I, Gasquet I, Kovess V, Le'pine JP. Prevalence and risk factors for suicide ideation, plans and attempts in the French general population: results from the ESEMeD study. Encéphale. 2012;38(4):296–303.
Nordström P, et al. CSF 5-HIAA predicts suicide risk after attempted suicide. Suicide Life Threat Behav. 1994;24(1):1–9.
Ozdemir E, Karaman MG, Yurteri N, Erdogan A. A case of suicide attempt with long-acting methylphenidate (Concerta). Atten Defic Hyperact Disord. 2010;2(3):103–5.
Polanczyk G, de Lima MS, Horta BL, Biederman J, Rohde LA. The worldwide prevalence of ADHD: a systematic review and metaregression analysis. Am J Psychiatry. 2007;164(6):942–8.
Santosh PJ, Sattar S, Canagaratnam M. Efficacy and tolerability of pharmacotherapies for attention-deficit hyperactivity disorder in adults. CNS Drugs. 2011;25(9):737–63.
Sharav VH. The impact of the Food and Drug Administration Modernization Act on the recruitment of children for research. Ethical Hum Sci Serv. 2003 Summer;5(2):83–108.
Shaw P, Stringaris A, Nigg J, Leibenluft E. Emotion dysregulation in attention deficit hyperactivity disorder. Am J Psychiatry. 2014;171(3):276–93.
Swann AC, Steinberg JL, Lijffijt M, Moeller FG. Impulsivity: differential relationship to depression and mania in bipolar disorder. J Affect Disord. 2008;106(3):241–8. Epub 2007 Sep 5
Wakschlag LS, Estabrook R, Petitclerc A, Henry D, Burns JL, Perlman SB, Voss JL, Pine DS, Leibenluft E, Briggs-Gowan ML. Clinical implications of a dimensional approach: the normal:abnormal spectrum of early irritability. J Am Acad Child Adolesc Psychiatry. 2015;54(8):626–34.

Other Suggested Readings

Achenbach TM, Rescorla LA. Manual for the ASEBA school-age forms & profiles: an integrated system of multi-informant assessment. Burlington: University of Vermont, Research Center for Children, Youth & Families; 2001.
Ambrosini PJ. Historical development and present status of the schedule for affective disorders and schizophrenia for school-age children (K-SADS). J Am Acad Child Adolesc Psychiatry. 2000;39:49.

Antshel KM. Psychosocial interventions in attention-deficit/hyperactivity disorder: update. Child Adolesc Psychiatr Clin N Am. 2015;24(1):79–97.

Arnold LE, Demeter C, et al. Pediatric bipolar spectrum disorder and ADHD: comparison and comorbidity in the LAMS clinical sample. Bipolar Disord. 2011;13:509–21.

Biederman J, Mick E, Faraone SV, Spencer J, Wilens TE, Wozniak J. Pediatric mania: a developmental subtype of bipolar disorder? Biol Psychiatry. 2000;48(6):458–66.

Biederman J, Petty CR, Byrne D, Wong P, Wozniak J, Faraone SV. Risk for switch from unipolar to bipolar disorder in youth with ADHD: a long term prospective controlled study. J Affect Disord. 2009;119:16–21.

Bond DJ, Hadjipavlou G, Lam RW, McIntyre RS, Beaulieu S, Schaffer A, Weiss M. Canadian Network for Mood and Anxiety Treatments (CANMAT) Task Force. The Canadian Network for Mood and Anxiety Treatments (CANMAT) task force recommendations for the management of patients with mood disorders and comorbid attention-deficit/hyperactivity disorder. Ann Clin Psychiatry. 2012;24(1):23–37.

Chang KD. Course and impact of bipolar disorder in young patients. J Clin Psychiatry. 2010;71(2):e05. https://doi.org/10.4088/JCP.8125tx7c. Review. PubMed PMID: 20193644

Correll CU, Kratochvil CJ, March JS. Developments in pediatric psychopharmacology: focus on stimulants, antidepressants, and antipsychotics. J Clin Psychiatry. 2011;72(5):655–70. https://doi.org/10.4088/JCP.11r07064. Review. PubMed PMID: 21658348

Correll CU, Hauser M, Penzner JB, et al. Type and duration of subsyndromal symptoms in youth with bipolar I disorder prior to their first manicepisode. Bipolar Disord. 2014;16:478–92.

Daviss WB. A review of co-morbid depression in pediatric ADHD: etiology, phenomenology, and treatment. J Child Adolesc Psychopharmacol. 2008;18(6):565–71.

Findling RL. Diagnosis and treatment of bipolar disorder in young patients. J Clin Psychiatry. 2009;70(12):e45.

Frías Á, Palma C, Farriols N. Comorbidity in pediatric bipolar disorder: prevalence, clinical impact, etiology and treatment. J Affect Disord. 2015;174:378–89.

Geller B, Zimerman B, Williams M, et al. Reliability of the Washington University in St. Louis Kiddie Schedule for Affective Disorders and Schizophrenia (WASH-UKSADS) mania and rapid cycling sections. J Am Acad Child Adolesc Psychiatry. 2001;40:450–5.

Jerrell JM, McIntyre RS, Park YM. Correlates of incident bipolar disorder in children and adolescents diagnosed with attention-deficit/hyperactivity disorder. J Clin Psychiatry. 2014;75(11):e1278–83.

Joshi G, Wilens T. Comorbidity in pediatric bipolar disorder. Child Adolesc Psychiatr Clin N Am. 2009;18(2):291–319, vii–viii

Judd LL, Schettler PJ, Akiskal H, Coryell W, Fawcett J, Fiedorowicz JG, et al. Prevalence and clinical significance of subsyndromal manic symptoms, including irritability and psychomotor agitation, during bipolar major depressive episodes. J Affect Disord. 2012;138(3):440–8.

Kowatch RA. Diagnosis, phenomenology, differential diagnosis, and comorbidity of pediatric bipolar disorder. J Clin Psychiatry. 2016;(77 Suppl E1):e1.

Leverich GS, Post RM, Keck PE Jr, Altshuler LL, Frye MA, Kupka RW, et al. The poor prognosis of childhood-onset bipolar disorder. J Pediatr. 2007;150(5):485–90.

Liu HY, Potter MP, Woodworth KY, Yorks DM, Petty CR, Wozniak JR, Faraone SV, Biederman J. Pharmacologic treatments for pediatric bipolar disorder: a review and meta-analysis. J Am Acad Child Adolesc Psychiatry. 2011;50(8):749–62.e39.

Liu CC, Lan CC, Chen YS. Atomoxetine-induced mania with auditory hallucination in an 8-year-old boy with attention-deficit/hyperactivitydisorder and ticdisorder. J Child Adolesc Psychopharmacol. 2014;24:466–7.

Masi G, Perugi G, Toni C, Millepiedi S, Mucci M, Bertini N, Pfanner C. Attention-deficit hyperactivity disorder – bipolar comorbidity in children and adolescents. Bipolar Disord. 2006;8:373–81.

Nandagopal JJ, DelBello MP, Kowatch R. Pharmacologic treatment of pediatric bipolar disorder. Child Adolesc Psychiatr Clin N Am. 2009;18(2):455–69, x

Perlis RH, Dennehy EB, Miklowitz DJ, Delbello MP, Ostacher M, Calabrese JR, et al. Retrospective age at onset of bipolar disorder and outcome during two-year follow-up: results from the STEP-BD study. Bipolar Disord. 2009;11(4):391–400.

Polanczyk GV, Willcutt EG, Salum GA, Kieling C, Rohde LA. ADHD prevalence estimates across three decades: an updated systematic review and meta-regression analysis. Int J Epidemiol. 2014;43(2):434–42.

Scheffer RE. Concurrent ADHD and bipolar disorder. Curr Psychiatry Rep. 2007;9(5):415–9.

Serrano E, Ezpeleta L, Castro-Fornieles J. Comorbidity and phenomenology of bipolar disorder in children with ADHD. J Atten Disord. 2013;17:330–8.

Taurines R, Schmitt J, Renner T, Conner AC, Warnke A, Romanos M. Developmental comorbidity in attention-deficit/hyperactivity disorder. Atten Defic Hyperact Disord. 2010;2(4):267–89. https://doi.org/10.1007/s12402-010-0040-0. Epub 2010 Nov 10. Review. PubMed PMID: 21432612

Taylor E. Managing bipolar disorders in children and adolescents. Nat Rev Neurol. 2009;5(9):484–91. https://doi.org/10.1038/nrneurol.2009.117. Epub 2009 Aug 11. Review. PubMed PMID: 19668245

Thomas T, Stansifer L, Findling RL. Psychopharmacology of pediatric bipolar disorders in children and adolescents. Pediatr Clin N Am. 2011;58(1):173–87, xii

Van Meter AR, Moreira AL, Youngstrom EA. Meta-analysis of epidemiologic studies of pediatric bipolar disorder. J Clin Psychiatry. 2011;72(9):1250–6.

Wagner KD, Hirschfeld RM, Emslie GJ, et al. Mood Disorder Questionnaire for bipolar disorders in adolescents. J Clin Psychiatry. 2006;67(5):827–30.

West AE, Pavuluri MN. Psychosocial treatments for childhood and adolescent bipolar disorder. Child Adolesc Psychiatr Clin N Am. 2009;18(2):471–82, x-xi. https://doi.org/10.1016/j.chc.2008.11.009. Review. PubMed PMID: 19264274

Wigal SB. Efficacy and safety limitations of attention-deficit hyperactivity disorder pharmacotherapy in children and adults. CNS Drugs. 2009;23(Suppl 1):21–31. https://doi.org/10.2165/00023210-200923000-00004. Review. PubMed PMID: 19621975

Yatham LN, et al. Canadian Network for Mood and Anxiety Treatments (CANMAT) and International Society for Bipolar Disorders (ISBD) collaborative update of CANMAT guidelines for the management of patients with bipolar disorder: update 2009. Bipolar Disord. 2009;11(3):225–55.

Young RC, Biggs JT, Ziegler VE, Meyer DA. A rating scale for mania: reliability, validity and sensitivity. Br J Psychiatry. 1978;133:–429, 43.

ADHD and TIC Disorders

11

11.1 Objectives

- Describe the prevalence and morbidity of Tics, TS and ADHD
- List examples of simple and complex tics
- Understand the use of rating scales used in diagnosis or follow up in patients with Tics or TS
- List some disorders that can be included in the differential diagnosis of motor and vocal tics
- Describe the management of TS, Tics with or without ADHD

11.2 Describe the Prevalence and Morbidity of TS and ADHD?

A tic is defined as a sudden, rapid, involuntary, non-rhythmic movement or vocalization.

Tics result from the movement of one muscle or group of muscles and are characterized by their anatomical location, number, frequency, duration, and complexity.

Tics are classified as either simple or complex. Simple tics involve one muscle group or sound, whereas complex tics are slower and more purposeful, involving multiple muscle groups or multiple sounds, words, or phrases.

Tourette Syndrome (TS) also known as Gilles de la Tourette syndrome is a childhood onset neurodevelopmental disorder characterized by multiple motor and at least one vocal tic, both present for greater than 1 year, with onset before age 18 years (APA 2013).

Prevalence of TS is estimated to be 1% of the world's population (Robertson et al. 2009).

TS is more frequent in males than females, about 3–4 times more frequent.

J. Sadek, *Clinician's Guide to ADHD Comorbidities in Children and Adolescents*,
https://doi.org/10.1007/978-3-319-45635-5_11

Prevalence for other tic disorders has been reported as higher than TS, with ranges from 4% to 50% of school-aged children (Linazasoro et al. 2006).

Provisional (formerly known as transient) tic disorder (less than 1 year) is the most common tic disorder, with a prevalence of 20% of school-aged children (Khalifa and Von Knorring 2003).

The most common comorbid conditions of TS include ADHD with prevalence rates of around 50–75% and OCD, with prevalence rates of around and 20–60% of individuals with TS.

A bidirectional relationship: 50–75% of individuals with TS also meet criteria for ADHD; 20–30% of individuals with ADHD also meet criteria for tic disorder.

Children with TS also have higher rates of developing comorbid depressive and anxiety disorders, behaviour disorders, learning disabilities, and developmental disorders (Shaw and Coffey 2014).

The presence of comorbid ADHD appears to be one of the most important determinants of quality of life and, in the presence of comorbid ADHD, the rates of other comorbidities (e.g., rage, symptoms of seasonal affective disorder, sleep disturbances and depressive symptoms) are significantly higher than in TS only patients and contributes to poorer psychosocial outcome and educational problems (Hirschtritt et al. 2015; Lebowitz et al. 2012; Cravedi et al. 2017).

Recent review suggested that behavioral difficulties in TS with ADHD were found to be associated with the combined or hyperactive subtypes and that comorbid ADHD was associated with a higher rate of developmental coordination disorder (14% in TS plus ADHD group versus 7% in TS without ADHD group). (Cravedi et al. 2017)

11.3 Give Examples of Simple and Complex Tics?

- Eye blinking is a simple motor tic
- Tapping or touching objects is an example of complex motor tics
- Throat clearing is an example of a simple vocal tic
- Repeating others' words/phrases is an example of complex vocal tics (Shaw and Coffey 2014)

11.4 Give Example of Rating Scales Used in Diagnosis or Follow Up in Patients with Tics or TS?

- The **Yale Global Tic Severity Scale (YGTSS)** is a rating scale used to "rate the severity of motor and vocal tics over 5 domains, including number, frequency, intensity, complexity, and interference of tics with daily life". The **Yale Global Tic Severity Scale (YGTSS)** is a rating scale used to "rate the severity of motor and vocal tics over 5 domains, including number, frequency, intensity, complexity, and interference of tics with daily life"

- It can also be used as a way to score the impact of tic-related impairment, such as academic, occupational, social, family functioning, and self-esteem
- It can also be used as a way to score the impact of tic-related impairment, such as academic, occupational, social, family functioning, and self-esteem (Leckman et al. 1989; Shaw and Coffey 2014)

Examples of other questionnaires or scales:

- Tic Symptom Self Report Scale
- Tourette Syndrome Severity Scale
- Parent Tic Questionnaire (PTQ)
- Hopkins Motor/Vocal Scale

11.5 What Disorders Would You Include in the Differential Diagnosis of Motor and Vocal Tics?

Compulsions in OCD, Choreiform movements in Sydenham Chorea, Myoclonus, Dystonia, Stereotypic movement disorder, or stereotypies in autism spectrum disorder, Pediatric autoimmune neuropsychiatric disorders associated with Streptococcus/ pediatric acute onset neuropsychiatric syndrome, Allergic rhinitis and conjunctivitis, and Chronic cough (Shaw and Coffey 2014).

11.6 What Are the Considerations That Are Taken into Account When Clinicians Decide to Treat Tics?

Some researchers suggested that the decision to treat tics should be made if they cause any of the following:

- Sustained social problems (e.g., bullying, social isolation)
- Social or emotional problems (e.g., reactive depressive symptoms)
- Functional impairment
- Subjective discomfort (e.g., injury or pain) (Hartmann and Worbe 2013)

11.7 What Are the Principals of Management of TS, Tics and When Comorbid with ADHD?

- Treatment is multimodal and includes psychosocial treatment and pharmacotherapy
- Treatment involves the separation of tics and comorbid symptoms
- Mild tics that do not impair daily functioning or cause significant distress, often only need support and active monitoring, and do not need to be treated

- Psychoeducation may reduce stigma and relieve distress. It is important to educate about TS and related comorbid disorders. This will help parents and teachers to understand the diagnosis and allows the child to gain self-esteem and self-confidence
- Cognitive-behavioural therapy is first-line treatment of children and adults with tics
- Specifically, habit-reversal therapy (HRT), which is a component of comprehensive behavioural intervention for tics (CBIT) (Shaw and Coffey 2014)
- In the case where behaviour therapy is insufficient, pharmacotherapy is recommended.
- When pharmacotherapy has been decided, monotherapy is initially recommended at the lowest dose with gradual titration
- In most cases, ADHD symptoms are more impairing than tics. Tics wax and wean
- Cochrane review concluded that Methylphenidate, clonidine, guanfacine, and atomoxetine appear to reduce ADHD symptoms in children with tics. Authors also mentioned that although stimulants have not been shown to worsen tics in most people with tic disorders, they may nonetheless exacerbate tics in individual cases. In these instances, treatment with alpha agonists or atomoxetine may be an alternative (Pringsheim and Steeves 2011).
- Some researchers concluded in their reviews that higher doses of dextroamphetamine resulted in worsening of tics, but therapeutic doses of dextroamphetamine and methylphenidate did not result in worsening of tics in majority of patients (Hartmann and Worbe 2013).

11.8 Describe Some of the Nonpharmacological Treatment for Tics?

11.8.1 Habit-Reversal Therapy (HRT)

- HRT is the most commonly used behavioural intervention of TS
- It has had success and shown efficacy in randomized controlled trials (RCTs) in children and adults
- It includes the following components
  - Awareness training
  - Competing response practice
  - Habit control motivation
  - Generalization training
- These components teach patients to notice their tics, often through their premonitory urges, and to develop a competing behaviour to inhibit or interrupt the tic
- Usually the competing behaviour engages "antagonistic muscles to the muscles required to perform the tic", and is performed for 1–3 min or until the premonitory urge ceases

11.8.2 Comprehensive Behavioural Intervention for Tics (CBIT)

- CBIT is another first-line treatment of tics, which includes HRT, as well as functional assessment and function-based intervention procedures
- It aids in reducing triggers in daily life that worsen tics
- According to research, CBIT and HRT are preferred modes of treatment over supportive therapy and psychoeducation alone in the management of tics in children and adults

11.8.3 Exposure and Response Prevention (ERP)

- Exposure and response prevention (ERP) is another behavioural treatment used to treat TS. Also helpful in obsessive compulsive disorders.
- ERP is based on the relationship between premonitory urge and tic
- ERP results in a reduction of tics, by having the patient suppress their tics for an extended period of time after the premonitory urge, thus interrupting the association between premonitory urge and tic (Shaw and Coffey 2014)

11.9 Describe Some of the Pharmacological Treatments for Tics?

11.9.1 Alpha-Adrenergic Agonists

- Alpha-adrenergic agonists are first-line drug treatment for mild to moderate tics because of their efficacy and low possibility of adverse effects
  - Clonidine and Guanfacine are the two most common alpha-2 agonists
    They both act via a presynaptic alpha-2 adrenoceptor mechanism, resulting in the release of norepinephrine
    Studies have shown that both drugs have shown efficacy in reducing tics in individuals with or without ADHD
    Guanfacine is often preferred due to its milder adverse effects (less drowsiness and sedation)
  - Common adverse effects include sedation, headache, hypotension, and upset stomach (Scahill et al. 2001; Serajee and Mahbubul Huq 2015)

11.9.2 Neuroleptics

Neuroleptics had been used in the treatment of moderate to severe tics
Typical (first-generation) neuroleptics/antipsychotics

- **Haloperidol** and **pimozide** are the only two drugs that have been approved by the US Food and Drug Administration for the treatment of TS in the US

- They are *typical (first-generation) neuroleptics* and *antipsychotic* drugs that are act via dopamine D2 receptor antagonism
- Adverse effects associated with typical neuroleptics include: Sedation, Depression, Weight gain, Hepatotoxicity and Extrapyramidal symptoms, e.g., akathisia and acute dystonic reactions, parkinsonism, rigidity, abnormal movements, and tardive syndromes (e.g., tardive dyskinesia and tardive dystonia) (Serajee and Mahbubul Huq 2015)

Atypical (second-generation) neuroleptics/antipsychotics

- These drugs may act via dopamine D2 receptor (as do *typical antipsychotics*), and also block serotonin receptors to differing degrees
- Risperidone, aripiprazole, quetiapine are some *atypical antipsychotics* that have been studied for the treatment of TS
- Risperidone is the most studied atypical antipsychotic for the treatment of TS
- Aripiprazole has a different action than other atypical antipsychotics. It is a partial agonist at dopamine D2 and D3 receptors and it is a partial agonist at serotonin 5-HT (1A) receptors
- Adverse effects of atypical neuroleptics include sedation, metabolic effects (e.g., weight gain and glucose intolerance, dyslipidemia), cardiac adverse effects and extrapyramidal side effects (Serajee and Mahbubul Huq 2015).

11.9.3 Other Pharmacological Treatments

Other medications options that were used include: *Benzodiazepines* (e.g., clonazepam), atomoxetine, tetrabenazine, topiramate, baclofen, Onabotulinumtoxin A injections (Botulinum toxin can be used to target localized and potentially dangerous tics) and finally, in case of medication resistance, deep brain stimulation (DBS) can be considered" (Hartmann and Worbe 2013).

References

American Psychiatric Association. Diagnostic and statistical manual of mental disorders. 5th ed. Arlington VA: American Psychiatric Association; 2013.

Cravedi E, Deniau E, Giannitelli M, Xavier J, Hartmann A, Cohen D. Tourette syndrome and other neurodevelopmental disorders: a comprehensive review. Child Adolesc Psychiatry Ment Health. 2017;11:59.

Hartmann A, Worbe Y. Pharmacological treatment of Gilles de la Tourette syndrome. Neurosci Biobehav Rev. 2013;37:1157–61.

Hirschtritt ME, Lee PC, Pauls DL, et al. Lifetime prevalence, age of risk, and genetic relationships of comorbid psychiatric disorders in Tourette syndrome. JAMA Psychiat. 2015;72:325–33.

Khalifa N, Von Knorring AL. Prevalence of tic disorders and Tourette syndrome in a Swedish school population. Dev Med Child Neurol. 2003;45:315–9.

Lebowitz ER, Motlagh MG, Katsovich L, et al. Tourette syndrome in youth with and without obsessive compulsive disorder and attention deficit hyperactivity disorder. Eur Child Adolesc Psychiatry. 2012;21:451–7.
Leckman JF, Riddle MA, Hardin MT, et al. The Yale Global Tic Severity Scale: initial testing of a clinician-rated scale of tic severity. J Am Acad Child Adolesc Psychiatry. 1989;28(4):566–73.
Linazasoro G, Van Blercom N, de Zarate CO. Prevalence of tic disorder in two schools in the Basque country: results and methodological caveats. Mov Disord. 2006;21(12):106–9.
Pringsheim T, Steeves T. Pharmacological treatment for Attention Deficit Hyperactivity Disorder (ADHD) in children with comorbid tic disorders. Cochrane Database Syst Rev. 2011;13(4):CD007990.
Robertson MM, Eapen V, Cavanna AE. The international prevalence, epidemiology, and clinical phenomenology of Tourette syndrome: a cross-cultural perspective. J Psychosom Res. 2009;67(6):475–83.
Scahill L, Chappell PB, Kim YS, et al. A placebo-controlled study of guanfacine in the treatment of children with tic disorders and attention deficit hyperactivity disorder. Am J Psychiatry. 2001;158:1067–74.
Serajee FJ, Mahbubul Huq AH. Advances in Tourette syndrome: diagnoses and treatment. Pediatr Clin N Am. 2015;62(3):687–701.
Shaw ZA, Coffey BJ. Tics and Tourette syndrome. Psychiatr Clin North Am. 2014;37(3):269–86.

Bibliography

Ganos C, Martino D. Tics and tourette syndrome. Neurol Clin. 2015;33(1):115–36.
Hallett M. Tourette syndrome: update. Brain Dev. 2015;37(7):651–5.
Schrock LE, Mink JW, Woods DW, Porta M, Servello D, Visser-Vandewalle V, Silburn PA, Foltynie T, Walker HC, Shahed-Jimenez J, Savica R, Klassen BT, Machado AG, Foote KD, Zhang JG, Hu W, Ackermans L, Temel Y, Mari Z, Changizi BK, Lozano A, Auyeung M, Kaido T, Agid Y, Welter ML, Khandhar SM, Mogilner AY, Pourfar MH, Walter BL, Juncos JL, Gross RE, Kuhn J, Leckman JF, Neimat JA, Okun MS, Tourette Syndrome Association International Deep Brain Stimulation (DBS) Database and Registry Study Group. Tourette syndrome deep brain stimulation: a review and updated recommendations. Mov Disord. 2015;30(4):448–71.
Serajee FJ, Mahbubul Huq AH. Advances in Tourette syndrome: diagnoses and treatment. Pediatr Clin North Am. 2015;62(3):687–701.
Smith H, Fox JR, Trayner P. The lived experiences of individuals with Tourette syndrome or tic disorders: a meta-synthesis of qualitative studies. Br J Psychol. 2015;106(4):609–34.
Swedo SE, Seidlitz J, Kovacevic M, Latimer ME, Hommer R, Lougee L, Grant P. Clinical presentation of pediatric autoimmune neuropsychiatric disorders associated with streptococcal infections in research and community settings. J Child Adolesc Psychopharmacol. 2015;25(1):26–30. https://doi.org/10.1089/cap.2014.0073. PubMed PMID: 25695941; PubMed Central PMCID: PMC4340334.
Yael D, Vinner E, Bar-Gad I. Pathophysiology of tic disorders. Mov Disord. 2015;30(9):1171–8.

Appendices

Appendix A: How to Diagnose ADHD in Children and Adolescents

1. Identify your patients: 3–18 year old patient identified with signs or symptoms suggesting ADHD. Symptoms can come from parents' direct concerns, or the mental health screen, or school, or other sources in group homes or institutions.
2. Review with the parents and patient their concerns, reason for referral, and the parents' and patient's (in the case of older children or adolescents) hopes for the assessment. Clarify if the symptoms have been present since the patient was young, and at what age they think the symptoms started, and how it progressed. Ask the parents, or patient, to bring all past documentation (e.g., school report cards, assessments, etc.). Obtain written consent to release information for institutional documentation. It is suggested that asking for documentation can be done by phone prior to the interview.
3. Obtain past psychiatric history and any prior ADHD diagnosis, medical history, family history of ADHD and other psychiatric and medical disorders.
4. Obtain the psychosocial history including pregnancy, birth history, developmental milestones, school performance, learning problems, parenting, abuse (both sexual and physical), temperament, relationship with others at home and at school, defiance and oppositional behavior, conduct related problems, and ask about current stressors and current medications.
5. Review of systems would include basic screening for comorbidities or presence of other disorders as mood disorder, anxiety disorder, learning disorders, sleeping problems, tics, seizure disorders, and substance abuse in adolescents.
6. Document that a physical examination was completed with an emphasis on hearing, vision, weight and neurological exam. Review routine blood work, including TSH. Ensure that there are no other medical causes of the symptoms of ADHD. Ensure that there are no medical contraindications to the use of medications for the treatment of ADHD symptoms.

J. Sadek, *Clinician's Guide to ADHD Comorbidities in Children and Adolescents*,
https://doi.org/10.1007/978-3-319-45635-5

7. Use rating scales and questionnaires (some are available at www.caddra.ca). SNAP is a free scale that can be used. It is an efficient way to obtain information from the patient and get collateral sources mainly from parents and teachers. They should be updated over time. Clinical judgment is mandatory for the interpretation of the results of these scales and questionnaires. Use the DSM-V criteria to verify if the patient fulfills DSM-V criteria, or not.

Appendix B: List of Scales: Children

- **Behavior Assessment System for Children (BASC):** This scale addresses externalizing and internalizing problems, as well as school problems. It has a behavioral symptoms index and adaptive skills index. (broad band).
- **Child Behavior Checklist (CBCL):** There are two forms of this scale, one is a parent completed and the other is teacher completed (TRF). It is available at www.aseba.org/index.html. (broad band).
- **Academic Performance Rating Scale (APRS):** The APRS is a 19 item scale for determining a child's academic productivity and accuracy in grades 1–6 that has 6 scale points; construct, concurrent and discriminant validity data, as well as norms (n = 247) available.
- **ADHD Rating Scale-IV:** The ADHD Rating Scale-IV is an 18 item scale using DSM-IV criteria. It can be completed by either parents (home form) or teachers (school form).
- **Brown ADD Rating Scales (BADDS):** It was first published in self-reporting format in 1996 for adolescents. It focused on the inattention and executive dysfunction not always apparent to observers. In the revised format different scales have been developed for different age groups, such as 3–7, 8–12, and 12–18 years of age, thus focusing on the symptoms of ADHD through the different development stages. Self-report format is available from age 8 and up, parent and teacher scales are available for all ages. The tools are available at: www.drthomasebrown.com/assess_tools/index.html
- BADDS includes five clinically derived subscales or "clusters": (1) Organizing, Prioritizing and Activating to Work; (2) Focusing, Sustaining, and Shifting Attention to Tasks; (3) Regulating Alertness, Sustaining Effort, and Processing Speed; (4) Managing Frustration and Modulating Emotions; and (5) Utilizing Working Memory and Accessing Recall.
- **Conners Rating Scale (Revised):** CPRS-R is a parent and adolescent self-report version; for teachers Conners Teacher Rating Scale—Revised (CTRS-R); for adolescents Conners Wells Adolescent Self-Report Scale. (broad band).
- **Conners Rating Scale Revised (CRS-R):** This is a parent, teacher and adolescent self-reporting scale, each being available in long and short format. There are also three screening tools that give the option of administering a 12 item ADHD Index or an 18 item Symptoms Checklist (DSM-IV), or both. This is considered a broad band.
- **Copeland Symptom Checklist for Attention Deficit Disorders—Child and Adolescent Versions:** This checklist designed in 1987 addresses ten key areas, including: emotional difficulties, peer relationships, family interaction issues, maturity level, distractibility, activity level, impulsivity, degree of compliance, attention-seeking behaviors, and cognitive and visual-motor achievement.
- **Home Situations Questionnaire—Revised (HSQ-R), School Situations Questionnaire—Revised (SSQ-R):** The HSQ-R is a 14 item scale designed for parent reporting to assess specific problems with attention and concentration

across a variety of home and public situations that most commonly occur day to day. It takes about 5 min to complete and is used with ages 4–11.

- The teacher version, SSQ-R is a 12 item tool that identifies frequency and severity of the child's behaviorial problems at school. The age range for this format is also 4–11 and takes 5 min to complete.
- **Inattention/Overactivity with Aggression (IOWA) Conners Rating Scale:** The IOWA Conners is a 10 item scale developed to rate inattention/overactivity ratings and separate them from oppositional defiance. This instrument was one of the first rating scales developed to evaluate children and adolescents with ADHD.
- **Swanson, Nolan and Pelham (SNAP-IV):** The SNAP-IV is a 26 item scale that reflects DSM-III criteria for ADHD. It also screens for other DSM diagnoses. The SNAP-IV-Revised (SNAP-IV-R) (using DSM-IV criteria) is and 90 item scale for use with children ages 6–18 and takes about 10 min to administer. It includes symptoms of oppositional defiant disorder (ODD) and aggression. It is available at www.caddra.ca.
- **SKAMP:** The SKAMP is a 10 item scale that measures impairment of functioning at home and at school. Separate subscales measure the severity of impairment of inattention.
- **Vanderbilt ADHD Scale:** This is a diagnostic tool for parents and teachers that rates 35 symptoms and 8 performance items measuring ADHD symptoms and common comorbid conditions. The parent version contains all 18 ADHD symptoms, with items assessing comorbid conditions and performance. The Vanderbilt Assessment Scale has two components: symptoms assessment and an assessment of impairment of performance at home, school, and other social settings. This rating scale is used by professionals to screen for ADHD, oppositional defiant disorder, conduct disorder, anxiety and depression in children. The parent rating scale version contains 55 items, while the teacher version has 43 items and focuses on behavior an observations at school. Each takes about 10 min to complete, is free on line and is suitable for ages 6–12.

Other Tests

- **Intelligence tests** are not required to diagnose ADHD but they can be used in some cases during the general assessment. Examples are the **Wechsler Intelligence Scale for Children (WISC) and Stanford-Binet test**.
- **Achievement tests** are also not required to diagnose ADHD but are designed to measure a child's current level of functioning with regard to specific academic subjects, such as reading, writing, and math. They may also test knowledge and skills. Examples are **Woodcock-Johnson III, Wechsler Individual Achievement Test (WIAT), Wide Range Achievement Test (WRAT)**.
- **Attention tests** may also be useful. There is a wide variety to choose from. Examples are the **Conners CPT II Continuous Performance Test II (Version 5 for Windows), Integrated Visual and Auditory Continuous Performance Test (IVA), Tests for Variable Attention (TOVA)**.

- **Executive functioning** that includes problem solving abilities (i.e., reasoning, planning, and organization), flexibility in thinking, and the ability to integrate feedback from others and abstract can also be tested. Examples include the **Wisconsin Card Sort Test (WCST)**. This test is not a mandatory part of ADHD assessment.
- NB: AACAP Practice parameter for the Assessment and Treatment of Children and Adolescents with ADHD compiled a list of scales that is very useful.

Appendix C: Sadek ADHD Checklist (SAC) ©

	Symptom of Inattention: Mnemonic: Details Off	Never	Rarely	Sometimes	Often	Very often
D	**DETAILS** often missed or makes careless mistakes *in schoolwork, work, other activities*					
E	**EASILY distracted** by stimuli *(e.g. noise, movement, day dream a lot)*					
TA	**TASK AVOIDANCE** *(that requires attention such as homework, forms)*					
I	**INSTRUCTIONS** missed because mind elsewhere Or not listening when spoken to directly					
L	**LOSE** things (e.g. Books, wallet, keys, toy, homework)					
S	**SUSTAINING attention** is problematic *(during reading, classes, lectures or other activities)*					
O	**ORGANIZATIONAL problems** *(messy, disorganized work, difficulty organizing time)*					
F	**Fails to FINISH** *activities, schoolwork, chores or duties in the workplace* or not following through on instructions.					
F	**FORGETFUL** in daily activities *(e.g. doing homework, remembering appointments, paying bills)*					
	Total adults 5/9					
	Total children 6/9					
	Symptoms of Hyperactivity Impulsivity: **Mnemonic: RAPID GIRL**					
R	**RUNS** about or climbs excessively in inappropriate situation/ or **Restlessness** feeling					
A	**ANSWERS blurted** before question is complete or blurt out rude comments					
P	**PLENTY of talk** in social situation or play					
I	**INTERRUPTS OR INTRUDES on others** (e.g. butts in conversations or games,)					

	Symptom of Inattention: Mnemonic: Details Off	Never	Rarely	Sometimes	Often	Very often
D	**DIFFICULTY awaiting turn** (e.g. waiting to speak in turn, waiting on line, adult can cut through traffic)					
G	**GOING non-stop** or cannot unwind and relax					
I	**IMPATIENCE** with prolonged seating (leaves seat in classroom or long meeting)					
R	**RESTLESS**: always fidgets or squirms (e.g. taps legs or fingers)					
L	**LOUD** or noisy					
	Total adults 5/9					
	Total children 6/9					

Appendix D: Key Diagnostic Symptoms of ADHD

Inattentive Symptoms

- Does not give close attention to details or makes careless mistakes
- Has difficulty sustaining attention on tasks or play activities
- Does not seem to listen when directly spoken to
- Does not follow through on instructions and does not finish schoolwork, or chores
- Has trouble organizing tasks or activities
- Avoids, dislikes, or is reluctant to do tasks that need sustained mental effort
- Loses things needed for tasks or activities
- Easily distracted
- Forgetful in daily activities

Hyperactivity or Impulsivity Symptoms

- Fidgets with or taps hands or feet, or squirms in seat
- Leaves seat in situations when staying seated is expected
- Runs about or climbs when not appropriate (may present as feelings of restlessness in adolescents)
- Unable to play or undertake leisure activities quietly
- "On the go", acting as if "driven by a motor"
- Talks excessively
- Blurts out answers before a question has been finished
- Has difficulty waiting his or her turn
- Interrupts or intrudes on others

Appendix E: ADHD Differential Diagnosis

The list is compiled by Maryanne Sadek, University of Ottawa

Conditions that can mimic ADHD	Symptoms or signs not characteristic of ADHD
Psychiatric Disorders	
Generalized Anxiety Disorder	Worry for six months or more that the person cannot control; lack of energy; anxious mood and somatic anxiety symptoms.
Obsessive Compulsive Disorder	Presence of obsessions or compulsions that interfere with level of function.
Major Depression	Episodic change from baseline, Depressed or irritable mood during an episode; suicide-related issues; low energy; psychomotor retardation
Bipolar Disorder I or II (manic or hypomanic episode)	Episodic change from baseline; psychotic symptoms; grandiosity; pressured speech; recent decreased need for sleep.
Psychotic Disorder (schizophrenia or schizoaffective disorder)	Psychotic symptoms
Pervasive Developmental Disorder	Qualitative impairment in social interactions, communication or odd eccentric behaviors
Oppositional Defiant Disorder	Defiant; loses temper; annoys others and is easily annoyed; spiteful or vindictive
Conduct Disorder	Presence of conduct disorder criteria e.g. aggression to people and animals; destruction of property; deceitfulness or theft; serious violations of rules
Substance Abuse	Urine toxicology screen confirms presence of substance. Signs and symptoms of intoxication or withdrawal.
Specific Learning Disorder	Testing and consultation with learning disorder specialist confirms presence of the disorder
Language Disorder	Testing and consultation with speech-language specialist confirms presence of the disorder
Personality Disorders	
Borderline Personality Disorder	Abandonment anxiety; daily mood fluctuations; suicidal threats or behavior; identity disturbance; dissociative symptoms or paranoid thoughts; chronic feelings of emptiness.
Antisocial Personality Disorder	Lack of remorse; lack of responsibility; lack of empathy, deceitfulness and aggression
IQ-related problems: Intellectual disability	Cognitive assessment confirms diagnosis
Gifted child	Explore if curriculum is not well matched to child's ability
Medication-related	
Mood stabilizers with cognitive dulling adverse effect	
Decongestants or beta agonist with psychomotor activation	

continued

Appendix E: continued

Conditions that can mimic ADHD	Symptoms or signs not characteristic of ADHD
General Medical Condition	Investigations confirm the diagnosis of the medical condition
Head Trauma/Concussion	Since underlying ADHD can increase risk for head trauma, it is important to look for timing of cognitive symptoms apparition (present before, or appeared or worsened after head trauma)
Seizure Disorders	Neurology assessment confirms diagnosis
Tic Disorder/Tourette Syndrome	Presence of vocal or motor tics
Hearing Impairment or Vision Impairment	Audition and vision evaluation confirms diagnosis
Thyroid Dysfunction	TSH levels indicate hypothyroidism or hyperthyroidism
Hypoglycemia	Abnormally low glucose blood levels confirms diagnosis
Severe anemia	CBC and anemia investigations confirm diagnosis
Lead poisoning	Lead blood level measurement confirms diagnosis
Sleep disorders	Sleep lab assessment confirms diagnosis
Fragile X Syndrome	Genotype confirms diagnosis
Fetal Alcohol Syndrome	Molecular genetic testing for FMRI gene confirms diagnosis. Possible presence of mental retardation.
Phenylketonuria	Blood test confirms diagnosis
Neurofibromatosis	Café au lait spots
Other factors	
Unsafe or disruptive learning environment	
Family dysfunction or poor parenting	
Child abuse or neglect	
Attachment Disorder	

Appendix F: Monitoring of Children and Adolescents with ADHD

- Physician follow-up is recommended one month after initiating treatment.
- Height, weight, heart rate, blood pressure, symptoms, mood, and treatment adherence should be monitored at follow-up visits.
- Monthly visits may be required until medication dosing and timing are optimized.
- When an acceptable regimen is determined, follow-up is recommended at least every three months during the first year, and two or three times per year thereafter to assess control of symptoms, treatment adherence, and the presence of comorbid conditions.
- Medication holidays are unnecessary unless adverse effects (e.g., decreased growth velocity) are a concern.

Appendix G: ADHD Medications

Methylphenidate-based psychostimulants
Methylphenidate short acting, tablets 5 mg (generic) 10, 20 mg (Ritalin®) Tablet Pill can be crushed Duration of action: up to 3–4 h Starting dose: 5 mg b.i.d. to t.i.d. Dose titration: 5–10 mg at weekly intervals Max. dose/day: All ages = 60 mg
Biphentin® Extended release (capsules can be opened and contents dissolved) Capsules 10, 15, 20, 30, 40, 50, 60, 80 mg Duration of action: about 10 h Starting dose: 10–20 mg daily a.m. Dose titration 10 mg at weekly intervals Max. dose/day: Children and Adolescents = 60 mg and based on weight: 2 mg/kg
Concerta® Extended release tabs 18, 27, 36, 54 mg Tablet needs to swallowed whole to keep delivery mechanism intact Duration of action: up to 12 h Starting dose: 18 mg Dose titration: 18 mg at weekly intervals Max. dose/day: Children = 54 mg Adolescents = 54 mg/Adults = 72 mg Maximum dose based on weight: 2 mg/kg
Amphetamine-based psychostimulants
Dexedrine® (5 mg tablets Short acting) High risk for diversion, abuse and misuse Duration of action Duration: lasts about 4 h. Starting dose = 2.5–5 mg BID Dose titration by 2.5–5 mg at weekly intervals Maximum dose per day for Children and Adolescents = 20–30 mg
Intermediate acting **Dexedrine® spansules** 10, 15 mg (cannot be crushed) Duration of action Duration: lasts up to 6–8 h Starting dose = 10 mg daily in the morning Dose titration by 10 mg at weekly intervals Maximum dose per day for Children and Adolescents = 40 mg
Extended release **Adderall XR®** Capsules 5, 10, 15,20, 25, 30 mg and can be sprinkled Duration of action Duration: lasts up to 12 h Starting dose = 5–10 mg daily in the morning Dose titration by 5–10 mg at weekly intervals Maximum dose per day for Children and Adolescents = 30 mg Maximum dose based on weight: 1 mg/kg

Extended release **Vyvanse ®** Capsules 10, 20, 30, 40,50, 60, 70 mg Capsule content can be diluted in water, orange juice and yogurt Prodrug that may decrease risk of recreational abuse Duration of action Duration: lasts up to 13–14 h Starting dose = 10–20 mg daily in the morning Dose titration by 10 mg at weekly intervals Maximum dose per day for Children and Adolescents = 60 mg Maximum dose based on weight: 1 mg/kg
Non stimulants
Strattera (Atomoxetine) Capsules 10, 18, 25,40, 60, 80, 100 mg Capsule needs to swallowed whole to reduce GI side effects Duration of action: Up to 24 h Starting dose for Children and Adolescents: 0.5 mg/kg/day Maintain dose for a minimum of 7–14 days before adjusting: Children = 0.8 then 1.2 mg/kg/day Max. dose per day: 1.4 mg/kg/day or 100 mg
Intuniv XR® (Guanfacine XR) Extended release tabs 1, 2, 3, 4 mg Pills need to be swallowed whole to keep delivery mechanism intact Duration of action: Up to 24 h Starting dose for Children and Adolescents: 1 mg q.d. (morning or evening) Maintain dose for a minimum of 7 days before adjusting by no more than 1 mg increment weekly Maximum dose per day: Monotherapy in ages 6–12 years = 4 mg Maximum dose per day: Monotherapy in ages 13–17 years = 7 mg When used as adjunctive therapy to psychostimulants in ages 6–17, maximum dose 6–17 = 4 mg Maximum dose based on weight 27–40.5 kg = 2 mg 40.5–45 kg = 3 mg Above 45 kg = 4 mg at bedtime

ADHD medication effect size

Stimulant medications = 1.0 and 0.4–0.8 in preschoolers.

a-Agonist medications, ER = 0.7

Atomoxetine = 0.7

0.2 = small effect size, 0.5 = moderate effect size, 0.8 = large effect size.

Reference: Southammakosane C, PEDIATRICS Volume 136, number 2, August 2015

Appendix H: Management of Adverse Events of ADHD Medications

Adverse effects of stimulant medications include decreased appetite, sleep disturbance, headaches, irritability, nervousness, stomach upset, abdominal pain, nausea, abdominal discomfort, weight loss, growth suppression, seizure, tearfulness, stuttering, dizziness, increased heart rate and blood pressure.

More severe side effects (rare) can include psychotic symptoms and sensitivity reactions that will require discontinuation of the medication.

Special consideration had been given to the impact of ADHD medications on growth, tics, seizure, cardiac events and primary active psychotic disorders and bipolar disorder.

Management of Side Effects

- **Cardiovascular risk**
  - In May 2006, Health Canada issued important safety information on ADHD medications and recommended that ADHD drugs should be started at the lowest possible dose, and increased slowly, as individual patient response to these drugs is known to vary widely. The recommendation also stated that:

  ADHD drugs should not be used if a patient has:
  Symptomatic cardiac disease;
  Moderate to severe hypertension;
  Advance arteriosclerosis, coronary artery disease; or
  Hyperthyroidism
  - Generally, ADHD drugs should not be used in patients with known structural cardiac abnormalities. Before prescribing an ADHD drug, it is important to be aware of whether the patient has:

  a family history of sudden death, or death related to cardiac problems;
  participates in strenuous exercise; or
  takes other sympathomimetic drugs
  - These are thought to be additional risk factors. In patients with relevant risk factors, and based on the physician's judgment, further evaluation of the cardiovascular system may be considered before starting on the drug.
  - American Heart Association recommends that before beginning therapy of stimulant medications, careful history should be obtained with special attention to symptoms, such as palpitations, syncope, or near syncope. Medications use, such as other prescribed and over-the-counter medications, should be determined. The family history should be reviewed with reference to the long QT Syndrome or other causes of sudden, unexplained death. Detection of these symptoms, or risk factors, warrants a cardiovascular evaluation by a pediatric cardiologist before initiation of therapy.
  - Patients who are considered to need long-term treatment with ADHD drugs should undergo periodic evaluation of their cardiovascular status, based on the physician's judgment.

  - Patients taking drugs for the management of ADHD should be advised not to discontinue their medications without consultation with their physician.
  - At follow-up visits, patients receiving psychotropic drug therapy should be questioned about the addition of any drugs, and the occurrence of any of the above symptoms. The physical examination should include determination of heart rate and blood pressure.
  - ECG is not routinely recommended before starting stimulant medications.
  - Risk of sudden death is found to be similar to the general population.
- **Growth and appetite suppression**
  - Treatment with psychostimulant medications may result in a reduction in both height and weight. On average, the reduction in height amounts to approximately 1 cm per year during the first 1–3 years of treatment and 3 kg less than predicted over a year period.
  - In the majority of cases, these effects are usually minor and the majority of patients fall within the 95% of the population. The small group that suffer from significant growth suppression usually show a dose dependent effect with doses over 1.5 mg/kg/day (given continuously) resulting in more problems; preschool children may be particularly vulnerable to growth effects.
  - Reduced caloric intake and suboptimal nutrition due to appetite suppression are the more likely causes of most growth suppression. Other hypotheses considered were the dysregulation of receptors in the growth system, effect of ADHD on growth hormone, prolactin and possible increase or decrease in growth related to ADHD itself.
  - Monitor growth (weight and height) closely and use the growth charts.

– <u>Simple strategies that might be helpful</u>:

Consuming additional meals, or snacks, early in the morning or late in the evening when the stimulant effects of the drug have worn off

Obtaining dietary advice

Consuming high calorie foods of good nutritional value

Changing the timing of the dose and/or meals

Consuming high energy snacks

If growth is significantly affected by drug treatment (that is, the child or young person has not met the height expected for their age), the option of a planned break in treatment over school holidays may be considered to allow "catch-up" growth to occur. Drug holidays can be planned. Current data does not support specific guidelines indicating what magnitude of height or weight gain deceleration should trigger changes in the treatment regimen.

In children, you can follow the medical criteria for referral to pediatric endocrinologist to consider growth hormone therapy in treatment of short stature, particularly if the height is more than 2 standard deviations below the population mean for the age, and a one year decrease of more than .5 standard deviation in height. Consideration should also be given to the mother and father's height.

- **Jaundice, signs of liver disease or biliary obstruction**
  - Stop medication immediately and seek the help of a specialist.
- **Agitation or mood disturbance**
  - Discern direct medication (emotional symptoms correlate with expected time of medication effect) as opposed to rebound effect (emotional symptoms occur later in day as medication expected to wearing off)
  - If medication effect, discontinue medication
  - If rebound effect, may add short-acting stimulant in afternoon
- **Psychotic symptoms**
  - New onset psychotic symptoms that develop during the course of treatment of ADHD should be carefully evaluated. Development of psychosis as a side effect of psychostimulant is rare, and in most cases, the impact of psychotic adverse events is mild and mostly self-limiting. Several guidelines suggest that caution would be appropriate when prescribing ADHD drugs to children and young people with a family history of psychosis, or past history of psychotic episodes. A full psychiatric assessment should be conducted to determine if the psychotic symptoms are primary or secondary. A determination of starting an antipsychotic should be made at that point.
- **Seizures**
  - Despite the thin evidence of ADHD treatment in children with seizure disorder, it is not a contraindication to treat ADHD in the presence of seizure disorder.
  - New onset seizure has been observed after starting a few patients on ADHD medications, and ADHD patients have been shown to have incidence rates of unprovoked seizures and epilepsy two or three times greater than non-ADHD children. After careful evaluation, some patients who had documented seizure may start an antiepileptic medication.
  - If seizures are exacerbated in a child or young person with epilepsy, or de novo seizures emerge following introduction of stimulant or Atomoxetine, another approach is to discontinue the drug and trial a different class.
  - It is important to rule out the possibility of substance abuse inducing seizure in patients with ADHD.
  - Some studies support the lowering of seizure threshold with the use of psychostimulants but other studies found no evidence for an increase in relative risk for either MPH (0.8) or Atomoxetine (1.1)
  - Fatal hepatotoxicity has been reported as an extremely rare event in young epileptic children with polypharmacy or inborn errors of metabolism, and the combination of Atomoxetine with antiepileptic agents that might increase the risk of liver toxicity. Requires close clinical monitoring.
  - ADHD symptoms in epilepsy may be improved by non-specific interventions, such as better seizure control, decreasing AED polypharmacy, reducing drug interactions, and switching to AEDs with fewer cognitive and behavioral effects epilepsy.

- **Sleep disturbance**
  - Some clinicians concluded from several studies that the effect of ADHD medication on sleep may be beneficial, at least in some patients, but further research with more subjects, and with a variety of medication, is needed. Many patients treated with psychostimulants complain of insomnia, so an approach to manage this problem is necessary. Clinicians should document sleep patterns and complaints before treatment to help interpret problems that may arise after medication has been prescribed.
  - Sleep hygiene, consisting of simple behavioral approaches that promote sound sleep (e.g., creating a restful environment and avoiding caffeine), is a primary approach for most patients with insomnia.
  - It might be helpful to look into shifting the dose to an earlier time or reducing an existing evening dose.
  - Atomoxetine may have an effect on sleep that is different from that of psychostimulants, including reduced sleep latency, but less efficiency. In a randomized, double-blinded, crossover trial, Methylphenidate treatment for children with ADHD caused more initial insomnia, but fewer awakenings compared with Atomoxetine treatment. Switching to Atomoxetine may be considered for patients who prefer it, or who do not respond to adjunctive interventions for stimulant-associated insomnia.
  - Melatonin 3–6 mg at least half hour before sleep can be used. Other pharmacological options include: Trazodone 25–50 mg HS.
- **Suicide**
  - First, assess the suicide as a separate issue. Determine whether the patient is expressing suicidal ideation, intent, plan or is there a history of chronic self-harm behavior as in a personality disorder. Evaluate if suicide developed after starting Atomoxetine (more risk) or psychostimulant medications. Suicide prevention should be the first priority over any other consideration. You can use a tool, such as the Nova Scotia Suicide Risk Assessment Tool, to determine the risk level and management strategy. It is important to document all your findings about suicide and communicate them to others involved in the care of the patient. Caution is required when prescribing ADHD drugs to children and young adults with a past history of serious suicide attempts or depression. Families and caregivers should be advised of the need to recognize any emergence of emotional change, or self-injurious thinking, and to communicate well with the prescriber.
  - Patients being treated with ADHD drugs should be observed for the emergence of suicide-related events. If they do emerge in treatment, consideration should be given to dose reduction and/or other changes in therapeutic regimen, including the possibility of discontinuing medication, especially if symptoms are severe or abrupt in onset, or were not part of the patient's presenting symptoms.
- **Headache** Typically self-resolves and use symptomatic care

- **Priapism** (rare) Medical emergency; discontinue medication
- **Tics**
  - Tic Disorder is not a contraindication for psychostimulant use; however, several patients may suffer from worsening of tics. Taking a history, and closely monitoring comorbid tics is needed. It is important to note that several literature reviews suggested that stimulants are adequately safe in patients with both ADHD and Tic Disorder since tics are naturally waxing and waning. It is often difficult to decide if worsening of tics is provoked by the ADHD medication. If no impairment, no action. If distressing, taper or discontinue stimulant medication and consider guanfacine ER monotherapy or augmentation
  - Treatment of both Tics and ADHD symptoms can be treated together by adding antipsychotic medication to the psychostimulant or Atomoxetine. The alpha-2 adrenergic agonist Guanfacine or Clonidine have been showing promise in the treatment of patients with ADHD and tic disorders.

Common Side Effects and Contraindications: Atomoxetine

- The common adverse effects associated with ATX include decreased appetite, drowsiness, abdominal pain, nausea and vomiting, dizziness, increased heart rate and blood pressure.
- Less common side effects include dyspepsia and mood swings. There have been three published case reports of severe liver injury in children and adults using ATX. These individuals recovered when the drug was discontinued. Suicide-related behavior (suicide attempts and suicidal ideation) has been reported in patients treated with Atomoxetine.

Appendix I: ADHD Medication Contraindications and Drug Interactions

Contraindications to Stimulants

- Treatment with MAO inhibitors and for up to 14 days after discontinuation
- Glaucoma
- Advanced arteriosclerosis
- Untreated hyperthyroidism or thyroid dysfunction
- Known hypersensitivity or allergy to the products
- Moderate to severe hypertension (untreated)
- Pheochromocytoma
- Symptomatic cardiovascular disease or with potential to increase the risk of sudden cardiac death (e.g., coronary artery disease, structural heart disease, cardiomyopathy, history of arrhythmia).
- Acute psychiatric episodes of mania or psychosis

Contraindications to Atomoxetine (Strattera)

- Treatment with MAO inhibitors and for up to 14 days after discontinuation
- Glaucoma (narrow angle)
- Advanced arteriosclerosis
- Untreated hyperthyroidism or thyroid dysfunction
- Known hypersensitivity or allergy to the products
- Moderate to severe hypertension (untreated)
- Pheochromocytoma
- Symptomatic cardiovascular disease or with potential to increase the risk of sudden cardiac death (e.g., coronary artery disease, structural heart disease, cardiomyopathy, history of arrhythmia).

Contraindications to Guanfacine XR (Intuniv XR)

Known hypersensitivity or allergy to the products

Precautions are advised for those with a history of bradycardia, cardiovascular disease, heart block, hypotension, and syncope.

Main Potential Drug Interactions for Psychostimulants

- Monoamine oxidase inhibitors are contraindicated
- SSRIs and SNRIs—possible increased risk of serotonin syndrome
- TCAs—amphetamines and methylphenidate may interact with TCAs by different mechanisms
- Antipsychotics (e.g. chlorpromazine, fluphenazine)—may reduce the effect of amphetamines
- Anticonvulsants—methylphenidate may increase the level of phenytoin, primidone and phenobarbital
- Warfarin—methylphenidate may increase serum concentrations of warfarin

Main Potential Drug Interactions for Atomoxetine (Strattera)

- Monoamine oxidase inhibitors are contraindicated.
- Inhibitors of CYP2D6 (e.g., paroxetine, fluoxetine, bupropion, quinidine)—may increase atomoxetine serum concentrations.
- Decongestants (e.g. pseudoephedrine)—possible increase in blood pressure and heart rate.
- QT prolonging agents (e.g. quetiapine, quinidine)—May affect QTc interval, consider alternatives.

Main Potential Drug Interactions for Guanfacine XR (Intuniv XR)

- QT prolonging drugs (e.g. quetiapine, quinidine)—since Guanfacine XR may cause a decrease in heart rate, concomitant use with QT prolonging drugs is not recommended.
- Beta-blockers—may increase risk of rebound hypertensive effect if guanfacine XR is stopped abruptly.

- Anticonvulsants—Guanfacine XR may increase serum concentrations of valproic acid. Carbamazepine, phenobarbital and phenytoin may decrease serum concentrations of guanfacine XR through CYP3A4 induction.
- CYP3A4 inducers or inhibitors (e.g. rifampin, fluconazole, ritonavir)—Inducers may reduce serum concentrations of guanfacine XR
- CYP3A4 Inhibitors may increase serum concentrations of guanfacine XR.

Source: Canadian ADHD Practice Guidelines 4th Edition, 2018, www.caddra.ca

Appendix J: Selective Serotonin Reuptake Inhibitors (SSRIs) Dosing for Children and Adolescents

Name	FDA approval	Initial dose	Titration	Maximum dose
Fluoxetine (Prozac)	≥8 years old with depression ≥7 years old with OCD	<12 years, 5 mg/day ≥12 years, 10 mg/day	5 mg daily	40 mg/day
Sertraline (Zoloft)	≥6 years old with OCD	<12 years, 12.5 mg/day ≥12 years, 25 mg/day	25 mg for <12 50 mg ≥12	200 mg/day
Fluvoxamine (Luvox)	≥8 years old with OCD	25 mg/day	25 mg (divide BID for doses >50 mg/day)	<12 years, 200 mg/day ≥12 years, 300 mg/day
Citalopram (Celexa)		<12 years, 10 mg/day; ≥12 years, 20 mg/day	<12 years, 5 mg; ≥12 years, 10 mg	40 mg daily
Escitalopram (Cipralex)	≥12 years old with depression	<12 years, 5 mg/day ≥12 years, 10 mg/day	5 mg for <12 10 mg for ≥12	20 mg daily

Appendix K: Assessment Measures Available in Public Domain Free of Charge

Depression and Bipolar Disorders

Center for Epidemiological Studies Depression Scale for Children (CES-DC)

Designed for ages: 6–17

This is a 20-item self-report depression inventory with possible scores ranging from 0 to 60.

Higher CES-DC scores indicate increasing levels of depression.

Available at:

http://www.brightfutures.org/mentalhealth/pdf/professionals/bridges/ces_dc.pdf.

Depression Self-Rating Scale for Children (DSRS)

Designed for ages: 8–14

The DSRS is an 18-item self-report depression screening tool. It should take 5–10 min to complete this tool. Children who score 15 and over on the DSRS are significantly more likely to have a depressive diagnosis. This measure can be accessed at:

http://www.scalesandmeasures.net/files/files/Birleson%20Self-Rating%20Scale%20for%20Child%20Depressive%20Disorder.pdf

Patient Health Questionnaire-9 (PHQ-9)

Designed for ages: 13 or older

The PHQ-9 is a 9-item measure developed for assessing and monitoring depression severity. Items are self-administered.

Scores of 5, 10, 15, and 20 represent cut points for mild, moderate, moderately severe, and severe depression, respectively. Available at: http://www.phqscreeners.com/

Child Mania Rating Scale-Parent Version (CMRS-P) New!

Designed for ages: 5–17

The CMRS-P is 21-item parent-report measure designed to assess mania in youths ages 5–17. The CMRS-P may be used as a screening or diagnostic tool, and to monitor symptom changes over time. Available at: http://www.dbsalliance.org/pdfs/ChildManiaSurvey.pdf

Anxiety

Self-Report for Childhood Anxiety Related Disorders (SCARED)

Designed for ages: 8 and above

This measure is designed to screen for anxiety disorders.

It consists of 41 items that measure general anxiety, separation anxiety, social phobia, school phobia, and physical symptoms of anxiety. Both child self-report and parent report versions of SCARED are available at: www.pediatricbipolar.pitt.edu under resources/instruments.

Revised Children's Anxiety and Depression Scale (RCADS)

Designed for grades 3–12

The RCADS is a 47-item designed to assess depression and anxiety in youth.

The subscales of the measure include: separation anxiety disorder, social phobia, generalized anxiety disorder, panic disorder, obsessive compulsive disorder, and major depressive disorder.

Both youth and parent versions of the measure are available in several languages.

Available at: User Guide: http://www.childfirst.ucla.edu/RCADSGuide20110202.pdf

Child version http://www.childfirst.ucla.edu/RCADS%202009.pdf

Parent version: http://www.childfirst.ucla.edu/RCADS-P%202009.pdf

Spence Children's Anxiety Scale (SCAS)

Designed for ages: 7–18

The SCAS is a self-report measure of anxiety for children and adolescents.

The SCAS consists of 45 items (38 assessing anxiety, 7 items assessing social desirability).

The subscales include:

panic/agoraphobia, social anxiety, separation anxiety, generalized anxiety, fear of physical injury, and obsessions/compulsions.

Available at: http://www.scaswebsite.com/index.php?p=1_6

Penn State Worry Questionnaire for Children (PSWQ-C) New!

Designed for ages: 7–17

The PSWQ-C is a 14-item self-report questionnaire designed to assess worry in children and adolescents.

The PSWQ-C can be used as a screening tool. Total scores range from 0 to 42, with higher scores indicating greater tendency to worry. Available at: http://www.childfirst.ucla.edu/resources.html

Generalized Anxiety Disorder-7 (GAD-7)

Designed for youth ages: 13 and older

The GAD-7 is a 7-item anxiety measure developed after the PHQ. Items are self-administered and can be utilized in youth 13 years and older. Cut points of 5, 10, and 15 represent mild, moderate, and severe levels of anxiety. The screener is quick and user-friendly, improving the recognition rate of anxiety and facilitating diagnosis and treatment. Available at: http://www.phqscreeners.com/

Other Free Measures available from Center of School Mental Health at: http://csmh.umaryland.edu/

Appendix L: Helpful Websites

American academy of child and adolescent psychiatry website, Families and Youth resource center

http://www.aacap.org/AACAP/Families_and_Youth/Resource_Centers/ADHD_Resource_Center/Home.aspx
American Academy of Pediatrics http://www.healthychildren.org/english/health-issues/conditions/adhd/Pages/default.aspx
Children and Adults with ADHD http://www.chadd.org
FamilyDoctor.org http://familydoctor.org/familydoctor/en/diseases-conditions/attention-deficit-hyperactivity-disorder-adhd.html
National Institute for Children's Health Quality http://www.nichq.org/childrens-health/adhd.
National Institute of Mental Health http://www.nimh.nih.gov/health/topics/attention-deficit-hyperactivity-disorder-adhd/index.shtml
National Resource Center on ADHD http://www.help4adhd.org
U.S. government (education rights): Department of Education http://www2.ed.gov/about/offices/list/osers/osep/index.html and http://idea.ed.gov/explore/home

MIX
Papier aus verantwortungsvollen Quellen
Paper from responsible sources
FSC® C105338

If you have any concerns about our products, you can contact us on
ProductSafety@springernature.com

In case Publisher is established outside the EU, the EU authorized representative is:
Springer Nature Customer Service Center GmbH
Europaplatz 3, 69115 Heidelberg, Germany

Printed by Libri Plureos GmbH
in Hamburg, Germany